The 30-Minute
PALEO
COOKBOOK

90+ Delicious Recipes
for Busy People

Stephanie A. Meyer

Photography by Marija Vidal

ROCKRIDGE
PRESS

Interior & Cover Designer: Regina Stadnik
Art Producer: Karen Williams
Editor: Natasha Yglesias
Production Editor: Matt Burnett

Photography © 2020 Marija Vidal. Food styling by Elisabet der Nederlanden. Author photo courtesy of © Eliesa Johnson.
Cover: Zucchini Noodle Pad Thai, page 58

ISBN: Print 978-1-64611-478-8 | eBook 978-1-64611-479-5

R0

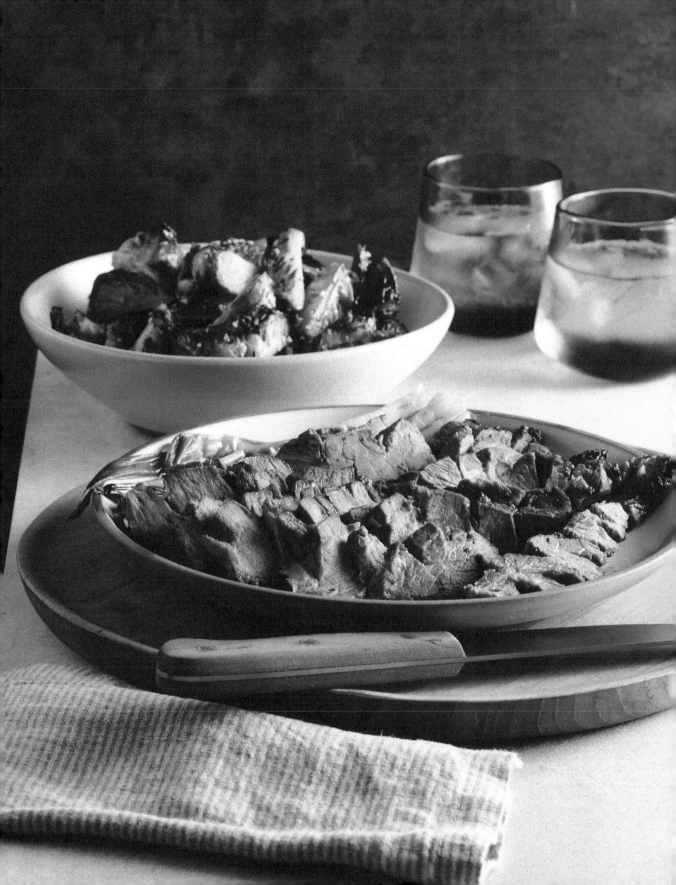

The 30-Minute
PALEO COOKBOOK

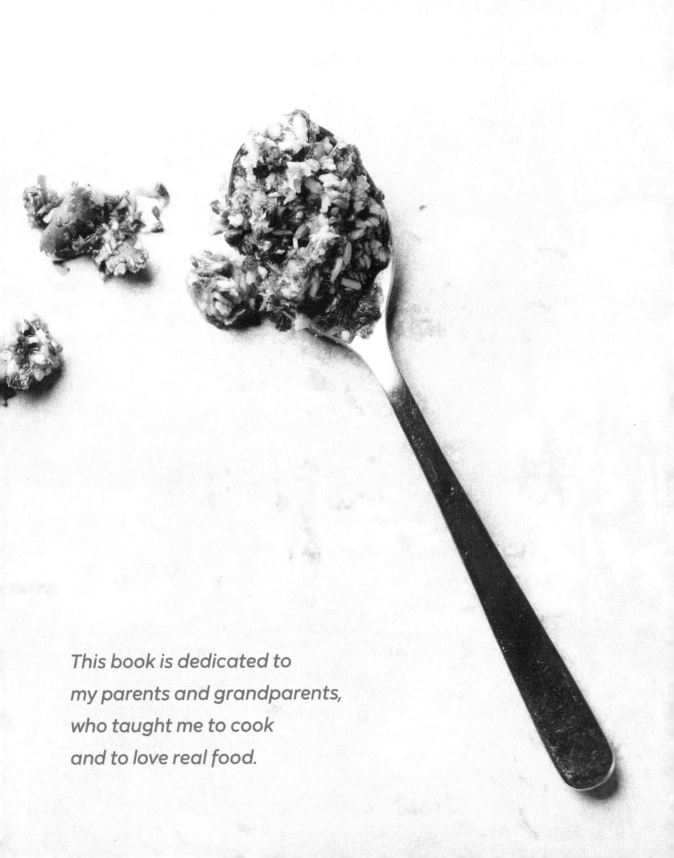

*This book is dedicated to
my parents and grandparents,
who taught me to cook
and to love real food.*

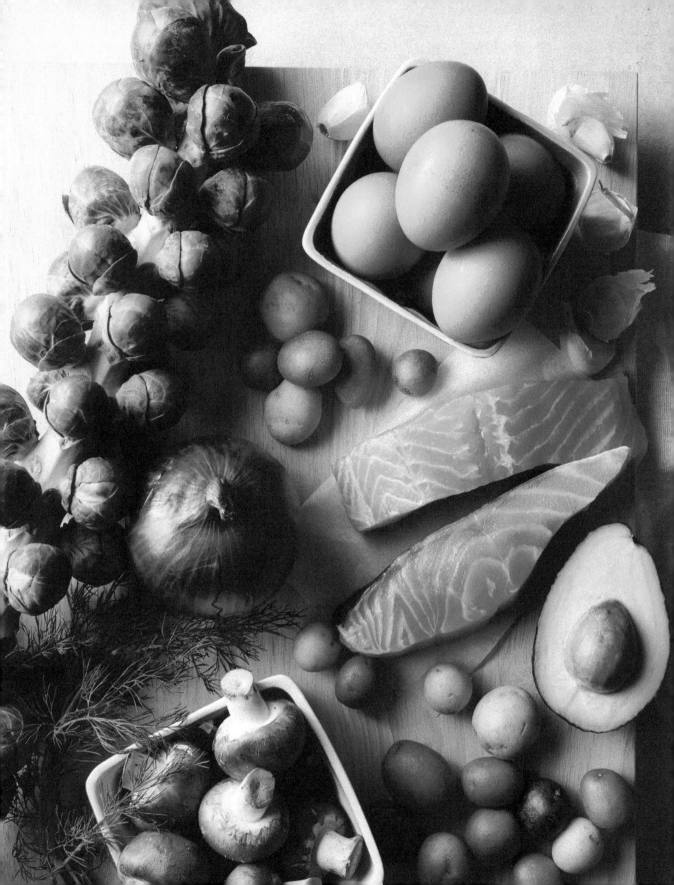

Contents

Introduction

For a good-size chunk of human history, finding anything to eat was an all-day challenge. It's modern humans who face the opposite problem: an overabundance of quick choices, many of which aren't particularly nutritious (processed, packaged, and fast foods) and in fact can be detrimental to our health.

So what's a busy, health-minded person to do? How do you eat well, but simply and quickly enough to make it happen consistently? After all, you'll see the health benefits of eating real, fresh food prepared at home only if you do it regularly.

I'm here to tell you it can be done. With modern tools and appliances, plus a collection of fast-and-simple recipes so delicious that you actually look forward to making and sharing them with your family, you can develop the habit of enjoying tasty, nutrient-dense meals at home.

My name is Stephanie Meyer, and I'm a cookbook author, recipe developer, writer of the food blog Fresh Tart, owner of a Paleo meal-planning company called Project Vibrancy Meals, and all-round Paleo cheerleader. I have been writing and sharing Paleo recipes for almost a decade, a journey that began when I was diagnosed with autoimmune thyroid disease in 2010.

I was lucky to be diagnosed by a physician who had experience seeing health improvements in her patients who eliminated gluten from their diets. I jumped right into a gluten-free diet, and then grain-free, as I began to experiment with uncovering food sensitivities and finding ways to feel better. Within weeks of adopting a Paleo diet, I noticed a decrease in my symptoms—facial swelling, joint pain, brain fog, bloating—and started to feel my energy return. Within a year, I was transformed. I lost weight, looked and felt like myself again, and had tons of energy—and my thyroid disease was in remission.

Adopting a Paleo lifestyle pushed my recipe development into new areas and introduced me to a whole new audience. I now have the pleasure of teaching classes and coaching clients, which allows me to talk face-to-face with people who are changing their health and their lives with quality food.

Paleo food is real food, and I'm very excited to share with you these 91 fast, simple, delicious recipes. I look forward to being in your kitchen with you as you make new favorite Paleo meals in 30 minutes or less. My goal is for you to reach for this book again and again.

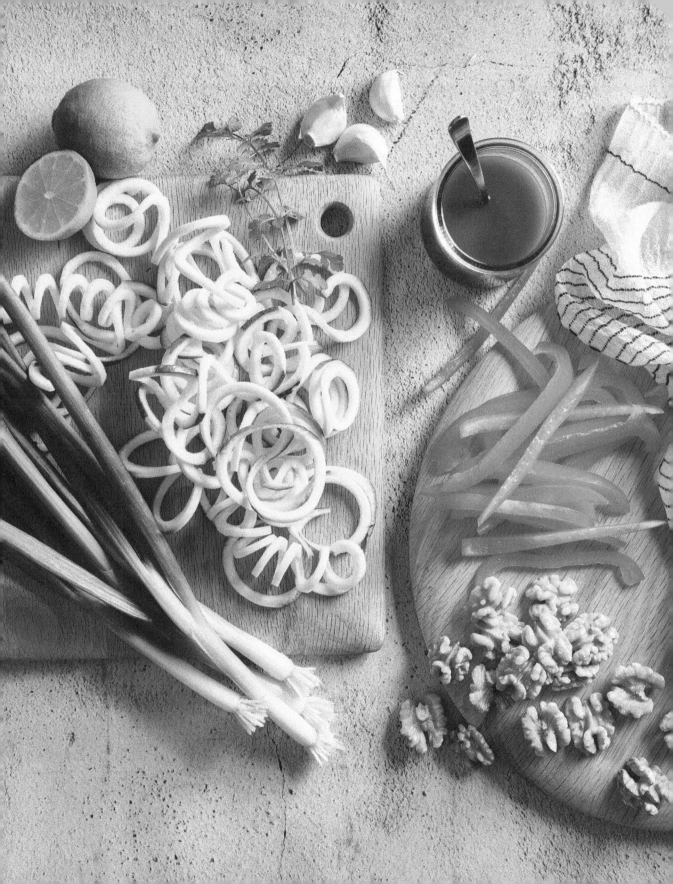

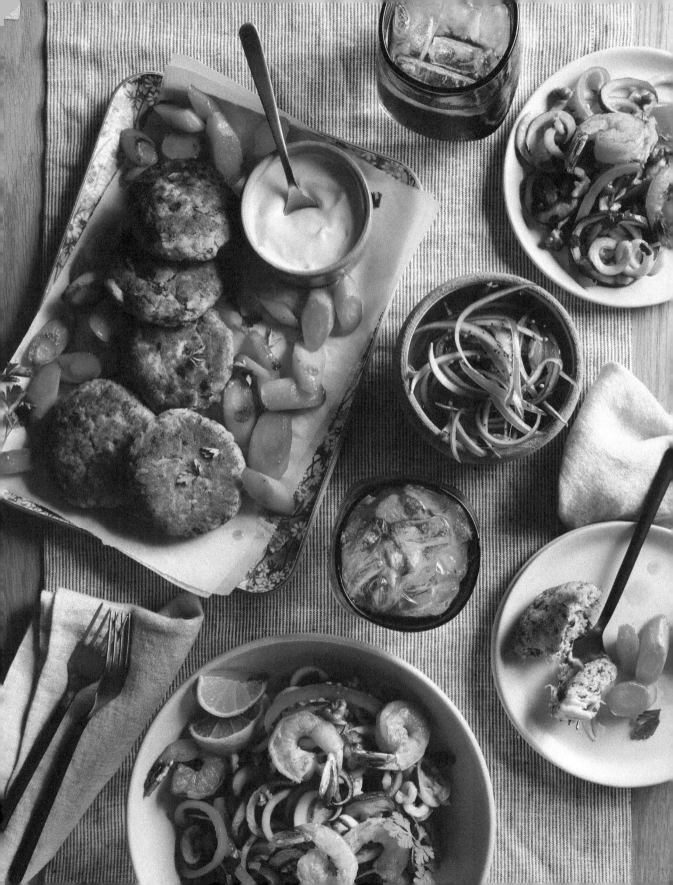

CHAPTER ONE

Caveman Principles, Modern Convenience

Let's get this straight right off the bat: Cooking real food from scratch doesn't have to take hours of preparation and cleanup. The packaged food industry likes to imply that it does, with clever marketing messages suggesting that we all deserve to be freed from the tedious chore of cooking, but it doesn't.

The truth is that with good tools, a little practice, and a book full of recipes like this one, you can prepare incredibly nutritious and memorable meals in as much time as it would take to order a pizza for delivery. In addition to enjoying the food, you can save money, trim your waistline, improve your health, and learn (and teach your children) an invaluable life skill.

And you can have fun doing it!

PALEO FOR THE REAL WORLD

While Paleo is often referred to as "the caveman diet," it makes more sense to call it "the real food diet." The term *Paleo* is short for *Paleolithic*, which describes eating the whole foods that humans evolved eating. The Paleolithic era predated agriculture, so the diet features what our ancestors hunted and gathered: meat, fish, vegetables, fruit, eggs, nuts and seeds, healthy fats, and the occasional honey. It doesn't include dairy products, legumes, or grains.

The Paleo diet was initially created as a healing diet, with the goal of preventing and treating chronic diseases that accompany a modern Western diet of packaged and processed food, including heart disease, diabetes, cancer, and Alzheimer's disease.

In the last decade or so, Paleo hit the big time when it became associated with weight loss and fitness. Nothing grabs the public's attention like before-and-after weight-loss photos! But while weight loss can be important, it's the healing aspects of a nutrient-dense Paleo diet that make it so powerful and why it's stood the test of time.

A healthy human body requires macronutrients (protein, fat, and carbohydrates) and micronutrients (vitamins and minerals) for survival. For instance, protein is used to build and repair tissues in our bodies. Healthy fats support vitamin and mineral absorption and brain function, and can help prevent heart disease and diabetes. Carbohydrates provide fuel and fiber for our bodies and brains, as well as our gut bacteria. And vitamins and minerals are used to perform literally billions of functions per second.

The Paleo diet, with its focus on the real food that humans evolved to eat, is both nutrient-dense *and* incredibly satisfying to eat.

The Challenge of Time

So, what does Paleo mean for you?

It means cooking simple, fresh food in your own kitchen and avoiding processed food. If that sounds daunting, I'm here to tell you that it doesn't have to be.

Most people don't cook at home because they think that they don't have time. And it's true that if you pick up a food magazine or start researching recipes online, you can find an abundance of recipes that can take hours—and most of the pots and pans in your kitchen—to prepare. When I was a young adult, this is exactly how I cooked. I read complicated cookbooks, made long grocery lists, and spent hours making dinner, leaving my kitchen a disaster and myself exhausted.

But I learned that it doesn't have to be that way. While it can be fun to prepare elaborate recipes for dinner parties and holidays, the daily routine of eating fresh, healthy meals at home comes from simple, no-fuss cooking. The beauty of the Paleo diet is that it's based on high-quality, nutritious ingredients that are delicious on their own.

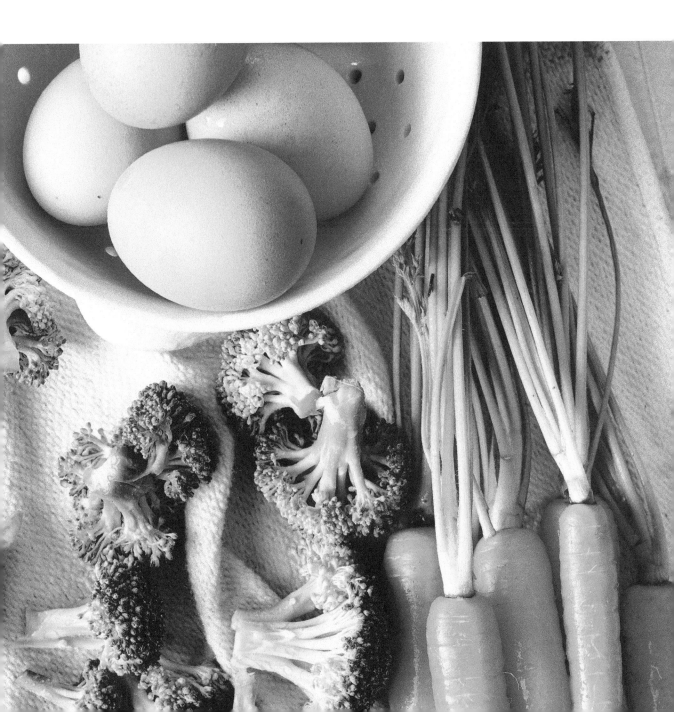

PALEO AT A GLANCE

Foods to enjoy on a Paleo diet:

- **Meat/Fish/Eggs.** Choose the highest-quality meats, fish, and eggs that fit your budget. When you can, go for grass-fed/wild/pastured versions of beef, bison, pork, lamb, chicken, turkey, game meats, fish, and shellfish and purchase pastured/free-range chicken and duck eggs.

- **Vegetables.** A Paleo diet is abundant in vegetables. All vegetables fit into a Paleo diet, with a particular focus on colorful vegetables.

- **Fruits.** All fresh fruits are Paleo.

- **Starches.** Sweet potatoes, potatoes, cassava, and plantains are all good sources of starch on a Paleo diet.

- **Cooking fats.** Avocado oil, coconut oil, and animal fats like lard, tallow, schmaltz, and ghee (clarified butter) are good Paleo fats to cook with. Extra-virgin olive oil and nut oils like walnut, sesame, or hazelnut oil are best eaten cold or only very lightly warmed. Sustainably sourced palm oil can be used for baking.

- **Nuts and seeds.** Raw, dehydrated, and roasted nuts and seeds make fantastic snacks in moderation and crunchy garnishes for soups and salads. Nut butters can be swirled into sauces and baked into cookies.

- **Sweeteners.** Natural sweeteners like maple syrup, honey, coconut sugar, molasses, monk fruit, and stevia can be used occasionally on a Paleo diet.

- **Flours.** Grain-free flours like almond (and other nut flours), cassava, plantain, arrowroot, tapioca, and tiger nut can be used occasionally on a Paleo diet.

Foods to avoid on a Paleo diet:

- **Grains.** This includes avoiding even gluten-free grains like rice, quinoa, and oats.

- **Dairy.** Avoid all dairy products, with the exception of ghee (clarified butter).

- **Legumes.** Legumes—including soy, peanuts, black beans, chickpeas, and lentils—are avoided on a Paleo diet. This includes flours and oils derived from legumes.

- **Industrial oils.** Avoid oils like canola oil, safflower oil, sunflower oil, corn oil, soybean oil, vegetables oils, vegetable shortening, and hydrogenated oils.

- **Packaged foods.** In general, I recommend staying away from packaged foods and snacks because they tend to be made with highly processed ingredients, sugar, and industrial oils. I include suggestions for high-quality Paleo products on page 13.

- **Sugar and artificial sweeteners.** White and brown sugar and artificial sweeteners like NutraSweet, Splenda, xylitol, and erythritol are to be avoided.

- **Alcohol.** Drinking alcohol is to be avoided on a Paleo diet since its active ingredient—ethanol—is a toxin. However, it is acceptable to cook with wine since the ethanol gets cooked away.

Paleo in 30 Minutes

I know that it's disheartening to come home at the end of a long day and not have options for putting a fast meal on the table. You may feel like you're far away from knowing how to look at a refrigerator full of fresh food and see meals instead of just ingredients. But in fact, you're about to acquire the essential life skill that's the difference between people who eat nutritious meals at home most nights and people who eat out most nights—and that life skill is simple cooking.

By picking up this book, you've acquired a cookbook full of recipes, of course, but you've also acquired a manual full of techniques that professional chefs and experienced home cooks use to streamline food preparation. While the meals are based on a Paleo template, the tools, equipment, and processes are very modern, and that saves time.

The meals in this book are designed for maximum flavor. It's a myth that a dish needs to be long-simmered with 20 ingredients to taste amazing. Most of the recipes that follow have 10 ingredients or less but don't skimp on the interplay of salty, spicy, bitter, tangy, sweet, savory, creamy, and crunchy that makes your favorite dishes memorable.

I've spent years keeping myself and my clients happy and satisfied with healthy, flavorful food that's fast to prepare. Soon you'll be doing the same for yourself and your loved ones!

COOKING FASTER: TIPS FROM THE PROS

1. **Maximize your microwave.** Defrost, reheat, parcook, and steam in the microwave to shave minutes off the prep time. Use your microwave to melt fats, cook potatoes, or even bake a mug cake.

2. **Use spice blends.** A collection of favorite spice blends can shortcut measuring and add fast flavor when you don't have time to chop fresh ingredients. Blends with citrus peel (like lemon or orange) can be extra flavorful; just make sure to include some oil to really bring out the flavors.

3. **Consider frozen options.** Frozen fruits and vegetables are nutritious and delicious and make life so much easier. Frozen berries, broccoli, and riced cauliflower in particular are often better than fresh. Frozen fish and shrimp can be defrosted quickly, which allows you to stock up and be prepared for quick meals.

4. **Skip the preheat.** Go ahead and get those veggies roasting! Unless you're baking, you can often pop food in the oven and use the preheat as cooking time, especially if you're cooking at lower heat anyway.

5. **Think small.** As in, cut food into smaller pieces. It can take 30 minutes to roast a whole sweet potato but only 10 minutes to roast a pan of 1-inch sweet potato pieces. When you're roasting dense vegetables, keep your dice small and dinner will be ready in no time.

The Convenient Paleo Kitchen

I have certain favorite kitchen tools (hello, Vitamix!), and once you get cooking, you'll quickly discover your own favorites and put them into heavy rotation. After a while, good tools feel like good friends you look forward to cooking with each day. Here are some recommendations.

MUST-HAVE EQUIPMENT

- **Sharp knives.** Arguably, the most important tool in any kitchen—restaurant or home—is a good sharp knife. Chopping vegetables with a dull knife is time-consuming and dangerous. Once you start working with truly sharp knives, you won't know how you got by without them. Choose an 8-inch chef's knife to get started; eventually add a good paring knife and you'll be in great shape.

- **Skillets.** You'll want at least two skillets, one 12-inch and one 10-inch. Nonstick is preferable for fast cleanup, although a well-seasoned cast iron pan is also very versatile. I work with both—a nonstick pan for cooking eggs and pancakes and a cast iron pan for browning meats and roasting food in the oven.

- **Saucepans.** Whether it's a stockpot or a Dutch oven, you'll need one large, heavy-duty pot with a lid for making bone broth and boiling vegetables and eggs. You'll also want a small or medium saucepan for smaller jobs.

- **Sheet pans.** Also called a baking sheet, choose a simple rimmed version in the largest size your oven can accommodate. I recommend buying at least two because you will use sheet pans for everything, from browning bacon to roasting vegetables to baking cookies.

NICE-TO-HAVE GADGETS

- **Pressure cooker.** An electric pressure cooker such as the popular Instant Pot is an excellent addition to a busy cook's kitchen. Use a pressure cooker to cook broths, sweet potatoes, chicken breasts, boiled eggs, and more in mere minutes.

- **Food processor.** I'm a big fan of Cuisinart food processors for their reliability and ease of cleanup. If your budget allows, choose a 14-cup version with attachments for slicing and grating. If you're short on space and funds, a mini-processor can be very useful for chopping vegetables and making pesto. A hand-held onion chopper is the most inexpensive option; it makes coarsely chopping onions and garlic super simple.

- **Blender/immersion blender.** I use my Vitamix blender every day, often more than once, for blending up smoothies, soups, batters, and nut butters. Of course, you can get by with a regular blender; read reviews online and find the model that's right for you. I also like an immersion blender to purée soups right in the pot, which saves time and cleanup.

SPEEDY PALEO MEALS

- **Eggs.** Whether fried, scrambled, boiled, poached, or baked, eggs are the perfect fast Paleo meal. Add sautéed greens and a snappy condiment and you've got a restaurant-quality dinner in minutes.

- **Go nuts.** Topping a simple salad or soup with nuts adds instant protein and healthy fat. If you don't have time to prepare a meal, a handful of nuts and a piece of fruit can keep you satisfied for hours.

- **Cook in bulk.** It makes all the sense in the world to cook extra food every time you cook. Stash the leftovers for lunch the next day or make a large batch of a protein and use it for more than one dinner. For example, leftover steak can be used in tacos on a second night and to top a salad on a third night. Or extra meatballs can be frozen for a future fast dinner.

- **Plan ahead.** Having a batch of bone broth and/or condiments like chimichurri on hand make it a snap to pull together soups, stir-fries, and skillet dinners.

- **Don't cook.** Instead, make a smoothie! It takes just minutes to toss fruit, greens, healthy fat, and protein powder in a blender and create a nourishing Paleo meal.

Time-Saving Ingredients

You can have the best intentions in the world, but if you don't have actual ingredients, home-cooked meals just aren't going to happen. Here is a list of staples to keep on hand.

PANTRY

- **Canned fish.** Canned tuna, sardines, and salmon are affordable, nutritious, and make terrific salads. Canned clams and bottled clam juice make fast clam chowder a possibility.

- **Sweet potato starch noodles (aka japchae or "glass" noodles).** Use these grain-free Korean noodles in ramen-style soups and stir-fries, or as a substitute for spaghetti.

- **Bone broth.** While packaged broth isn't as delicious or nutritious as homemade, in a pinch it can be used to create fast soups and pan sauces.

- **Apple cider vinegar.** Adding a touch of acid at the end of cooking a dish is often as important as adding salt. I think of apple cider vinegar as my secret ingredient for brightening gravies and stews, and of course it makes a classic vinaigrette.

- **Honey.** Raw honey is a nutritious food, as well as being a beloved sweetener. Honey whisked with vinegar or lemon juice makes a simple finishing sauce for sheet-pan dinners. Use honey to sweeten smoothies and breakfast porridges, as well as no-cook desserts like chocolate avocado pudding.

- **Canned tomatoes.** I like to keep an assortment of canned tomato products in the pantry: tomato paste, tomato sauce, whole tomatoes, and crushed tomatoes. From making classic spaghetti sauce to soups, a can of tomatoes is full of possibilities.

- **Nut and seed butters.** Don't stop at almond butter—cashew butter, tahini (sesame butter), sunflower seed butter, and even walnut butter are all readily available at grocery stores and add healthy fat, creaminess, and complexity to meals with no effort.

- **Collagen peptides.** Collagen peptides are derived from gelatin and are a flavorless, easy-to-dissolve form of protein. Collagen is the protein that makes bone broth so good for gut health and skin. Add these to smoothies, meatballs, puddings, soups, and even pancakes for a protein boost.

REFRIGERATOR

- **Mayonnaise.** Look for Paleo mayo made with avocado oil. Choose regular and/or spicy versions and combine with canned fish or chopped boiled eggs for diner-style salads.

- **Fish sauce.** Thai-style fish sauce is an umami-bomb that can elevate almost any savory dish to something special. Use a splash in sauces, gravies, salad dressings, and of course Asian-style coconut curries.

- **Dijon mustard.** I add Dijon mustard to most vinaigrettes, or combine it with mayonnaise for a quick dipping sauce for vegetables or creamy salad dressing. Add it to chicken and pork marinades for big flavor.

- **Capers.** Salty, tangy capers add fast zing to tuna and egg salads—or any salad, really—without requiring any chopping. Use them wherever olives would taste great.

- **Maple syrup.** Real maple syrup is my go-to sweetener for its depth of flavor, ease of pouring, and ability to hold its sweetness even when heated (unlike honey).

- **Coconut aminos.** If you're worried that you'll miss soy sauce on a Paleo diet, let me introduce you to coconut aminos, which is a liquid made from the aged sap of coconut flowers and salt. Coconut aminos is a terrific substitute for soy sauce, and many find that they prefer the taste, which has a hint of sweetness and a bit less saltiness than traditional soy sauce. It's terrific as a dipping sauce or as an ingredient in marinades and salad dressings.

FREEZER

- **Frozen fruit.** Toss into smoothies, heat with maple syrup for pancakes, or bake into a fruit crisp. Frozen berries and cherries in particular are cheaper than their fresh counterparts and always taste great. If your budget allows it, look for organic.

- **Wild shrimp and salmon.** Since I live in the Midwest, I tend to buy frozen fish. It's fresher than what I can purchase at a fish counter, and I can keep it on hand for fast meals. Individually packaged salmon fillets or peeled, deveined shrimp can defrost in minutes in a bowl of cold water.

- **Greens.** Add frozen kale or spinach to smoothies or sauté a few handfuls in extra-virgin olive oil with garlic. Top with a fried egg and you have dinner in 10 minutes.

- **Hash browns.** Look for a brand that contains just shredded potatoes. They brown quickly in avocado oil—or bacon fat—and can be the base for reheated leftovers or eggs.

- **Sausage.** I buy high-quality bulk sausage from my butcher and freeze it in patties. Add them to a pan as-is or simmer in a tomato sauce or soup.

FAVORITE PALEO BRANDS

When you're short on time but seeking big flavors, Paleo products can be a lifesaver. The number and quality of Paleo convenience foods and condiments has skyrocketed in the last couple of years, so you're starting Paleo at a great time. Many of these products are available at Whole Foods Market and well-stocked supermarkets; others must be ordered online. Here are my favorite brands:

- **Primal Kitchen.** Primal Kitchen uses best-quality ingredients in their mayo, ketchup, avocado oil, and salad dressings.
- **EPIC.** Known for their nose-to-tail philosophy, EPIC makes bone broth, energy bars, and truly craveable pork rind snacks.
- **Kettle & Fire.** I always prefer homemade bone broth for superior flavor, but in a pinch, I turn to Kettle & Fire bone broth.
- **Wild Planet.** Wild Planet offers a line of sustainably caught canned tuna, sardines, anchovies, and salmon.
- **Bob's Red Mill.** When you're shopping for dependably high-quality grain-free flours like almond, tapioca, arrowroot, and coconut, look no further than Bob's.
- **Otto's Naturals.** Otto's is a popular and trusted brand of cassava flour, which is the Paleo flour closest to wheat flour. It stands in beautifully in baked goods, pancakes, and crepes and can be used to thicken gravies and to bread foods before frying.

Continued >

- **Siete Foods.** With tortillas and tortilla chips made from almonds, coconut, and cassava, tacos and nachos are back on the menu.

- **Vital Proteins.** Vital Proteins sources from grass-fed and wild animals to make their collagen peptides powder, as well as other Paleo protein supplements.

- **Primal Palate.** Finding Paleo spice blends can be tricky, but Primal Palate makes it easy. From taco seasoning to pumpkin pie spice and everything in between, their blends are consistently fresh and always Paleo.

- **California Olive Ranch.** The olive oil business is rife with fraud, but California Olive Ranch always passes the test for pure extra-virgin olive oil. It's also delicious.

- **Hu Kitchen.** Hu chocolate bars are utterly amazing and will soon be your favorite treat. Guaranteed.

ABOUT THE RECIPES

You already know that the recipes in this book (except for a couple of staples) take 30 minutes or less to prep and cook, but here are some more ways that they'll help you make quick, easy meals.

- **Time-saving labels.** Many recipes have built-in shortcuts for those days when you really need to get a meal prepped quickly and easily. Look for these labels: 5 Ingredients (not including pantry staples like oil, vinegar, dried herbs and spices, etc.), No-Cook, One-Pan, Super Fast (10 minutes or less!).

- **Dietary labels.** You'll also see labels to help you quickly identify recipes that are Vegetarian, Vegan, Low-Carb (30 or fewer grams of carbohydrate per serving), and Nut-Free.

- **Tips that make recipes even easier.** Many recipes feature pro tips to help streamline meal planning and prep, such as ingredient swaps, cooking hacks, technique tricks, smart shopping ideas, serving suggestions, and optional flavor enhancements.

- **Foods to make in bulk.** Recipes for foods that store well, either in the refrigerator or freezer, include a note about making a bigger batch and stashing food for future fast meals.

All of the recipes are designed with speed, ease, *and* flavor in mind. These recipes borrow seasonings, techniques, ingredients, and flavors from all over the world. I'm excited to share all these exciting dishes with you!

It's also important to know that these recipes are nutrient-dense. Perhaps, like me, you've arrived at a Paleo diet to help manage your health. Our bodies need the nutrients in real food to function optimally, and these recipes will help you bring a wide variety of nutritious foods into your diet. Because Paleo food is whole, fresh food, it can help you better manage blood sugar, calorie intake, inflammation, appetite, and energy levels. Each meal is designed to provide you with adequate protein, healthy fat, and carbohydrates, so you are left feeling nourished and satisfied.

Paleo cooking is exciting cooking. Working with fresh, high-quality ingredients is a chef's dream come true and the same will be true for you. Once you get the hang of putting together simple Paleo meals, you'll look at farmers' markets and grocery stores in a whole new way. Instead of seeing ingredients, you'll see beautiful, abundant meals. Let's dig in.

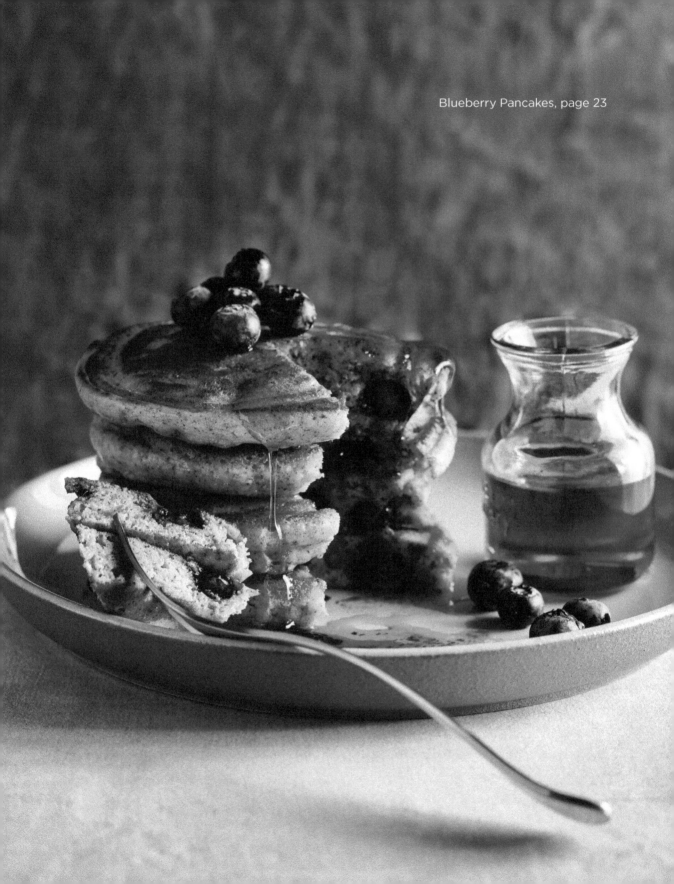

Blueberry Pancakes, page 23

CHAPTER TWO

Breakfast

Pork and Apple Patties with Maple Greens

Pork and greens are a well-loved pairing and make a deeply nutritious—and delicious!—start to the day. Feel free to serve alongside fruit or a fried egg.

SERVES 4

Active time: 20 minutes
Total time: 30 minutes

....

LOW-CARB, NUT-FREE

FOR THE PORK PATTIES

1 pound ground pork

1 tablespoon maple syrup

1 tablespoon rubbed sage

2 teaspoons arrowroot starch

1 teaspoon sea salt

¼ teaspoon ground nutmeg or mace

Freshly ground black pepper

2 bacon slices, finely chopped

1 cup chopped Swiss chard leaves, center ribs removed

1 apple, peeled, cored, and finely chopped

2 scallions, white and green parts, minced

FOR THE GREENS

1 to 2 teaspoons extra-virgin olive oil (as needed)

8 cups 1-inch pieces Swiss chard leaves, center ribs removed

2 teaspoons maple syrup

Sea salt

Freshly ground black pepper

1. **Get ready.** Preheat the oven to 375°F. Line a rimmed baking sheet with parchment paper or aluminum foil.

2. **Prepare the pork patties.** In a large mixing bowl, combine the pork, maple syrup, sage, arrowroot, salt, nutmeg, and several grinds of black pepper. Using your hands, mix gently until the seasonings are evenly incorporated. Set aside.

3. **Cook the pork patties.** In a 12-inch nonstick skillet, fry the bacon over medium heat until the fat is rendered but the bacon is not browned, about 5 minutes. Using a slotted spoon, transfer the bacon to a paper towel–lined plate to drain (leaving the drippings in the pan). Return the skillet to the heat. Add the chard, apple, and scallions, sprinkle with a pinch of salt, and cook until wilted, about 4 minutes. Using a slotted spoon, transfer the chard mixture to the pork; reserve the skillet. Add the bacon to the pork and, using your hands, gently mix to combine. Form the mixture into 8 equal patties,

setting them on the prepared baking sheet as you go. Bake the patties for 20 minutes.

4. **Cook the greens.** Meanwhile, return the skillet to medium heat. If the pan is dry, add the olive oil. Add the chard and maple syrup and cook for 3 minutes. Stir, then cover and cook for 3 more minutes. Uncover and cook, stirring, until wilted and tender, another 3 to 4 minutes. Season with salt and pepper. Serve the patties and greens together.

LOVE YOUR LEFTOVERS: These patties freeze very well, so consider doubling the recipe. Cool the patties to room temperature, put them in a zip-top bag with squares of parchment paper between them, and freeze. Reheat in a 350°F oven or skillet.

SIMPLE SWAP: You can substitute ground chicken for the ground pork.

Per Serving: *Calories: 475; Fat: 31g; Protein: 33g; Total Carbs: 16g; Fiber: 3g; Sodium: 319mg; Iron: 3mg*

Banana-Nut Smoothie Bowl

What's not to love about a smoothie that tastes like ice cream but is low in sugar and loaded with nutrients? The cold creaminess comes from a combination of frozen bananas, frozen cauliflower (you can't taste it, I swear!), and avocado.

SERVES 1 TO 2

Active time: 10 minutes
Total time: 10 minutes

NO-COOK, ONE-PAN, SUPER FAST

FOR THE SMOOTHIE BOWL

1 frozen peeled banana

1 cup packed fresh spinach

¼ cup frozen blueberries

¼ cup frozen cauliflower florets or cauliflower rice

½ avocado, pitted and peeled

½ cup water

1 tablespoon nut butter or sunflower seed butter

Maple syrup or stevia drops (optional)

Pinch sea salt

2 scoops (20g, or 2 heaping tablespoons) collagen peptides

FOR THE OPTIONAL TOPPINGS

Chopped nuts

Toasted sunflower seeds or pepitas

Chia seeds

Hemp seeds

Raspberries

Sliced strawberries

Sliced kiwi

Paleo chocolate chips

1. **Make the smoothie bowl.** Combine the banana, spinach, blueberries, cauliflower, avocado, water, nut butter, maple syrup (if using), and salt to a blender. Start blending on low speed, using a tamper if needed to break everything down. Slowly increase the speed, continuing to use the tamper, until very smooth, like soft-serve ice cream. Add the collagen and blend on low until just incorporated.

2. **Serve.** Pour into a bowl and add toppings as you like.

SIMPLE SWAP: Feel free to use ½ cup of frozen spinach or kale in place of the fresh spinach.

Per Serving *(1 smoothie bowl without toppings): Calories: 417; Fat: 19g; Protein: 24g; Total Carbs: 47g; Fiber: 13g; Sodium: 319mg; Iron: 2mg*

Grain-Free Porridge

When I was growing up in North Dakota (brrr!), warm, creamy porridges were my favorite breakfast. I loved to stir in lots of crunchy nuts and seeds, so it wasn't a huge leap to just *make* the porridge from nuts and seeds. Don't skip the flaxseed meal, coconut flour, or chia seeds—together they create the smooth thickness of a true porridge.

SERVES 2

Active time: 10 minutes
Total time: 10 minutes

. . . .

LOW-CARB, SUPER FAST

FOR THE PORRIDGE

¼ cup flaked unsweetened coconut

2 tablespoons raw or toasted walnuts

2 tablespoons raw or toasted cashews

2 tablespoons flaxseed meal

2 tablespoons coconut flour

1 tablespoon chia seeds

1 teaspoon pumpkin pie spice

1 cup unsweetened almond milk

2 scoops collagen peptides

1 tablespoon maple syrup

¼ teaspoon sea salt

FOR THE OPTIONAL TOPPINGS

2 teaspoons ghee or coconut oil

½ cup raspberries or blueberries

Maple syrup or raw honey

Warm full-fat coconut milk

1. **Prepare the porridge.** Combine the coconut, walnuts, and cashews in a food processor. Pulse several times until the mixture is chopped but still has texture. Add the flaxseed meal, coconut flour, chia seeds, and pumpkin pie spice and pulse once or twice, just to combine. Set aside.

2. **Make the porridge.** Combine the almond milk, collagen, maple syrup, and salt in a medium saucepan and set over medium heat. When the milk is steaming (it doesn't have to boil), remove the pan from the heat and stir in the porridge mixture until smooth.

3. **Serve.** Divide the porridge between two bowls and add toppings as you like.

SIMPLE SWAP: Substitute ripe peaches or pears or 2 tablespoons of raisins for the berries.

Per Serving *(without toppings): Calories: 425; Fat: 31g; Protein: 15g; Total Carbs: 27g; Fiber: 7g; Sodium: 393mg; Iron: 4mg*

PB&J Granola Parfaits

If you find yourself missing peanut butter and jelly sandwiches, this parfait is for you. Nutty grain-free granola, strawberry jam, and bananas are layered into coconut yogurt for a low-sugar breakfast treat that could also be served as a healthy dessert. What's not to love? To boost the protein, stir 4 scoops of collagen peptides into the yogurt before making the parfaits.

SERVES 4

Active time: 10 minutes
Total time: 10 minutes

5 INGREDIENTS, NO-COOK,
ONE-PAN, SUPER FAST, VEGAN

4 cups plain coconut yogurt

8 teaspoons no-sugar-added
strawberry or raspberry jam

2 bananas, cut into 16 slices each

1 cup Warm-Spice Granola (page 162)
or store-bought Paleo granola

1. **Prepare.** Set out four large glasses or cereal bowls.

2. **Make the parfaits.** Spoon ½ cup of yogurt into the bottom of each glass. Top each with 1 teaspoon of jam. Add 4 banana slices to each glass. Sprinkle with 2 tablespoons of granola.

3. **Finish.** Repeat, layering the remaining yogurt, jam, banana slices, and granola. Serve immediately.

Per Serving: *Calories: 383; Fat: 16g; Protein: 3g; Total Carbs: 54g; Fiber: 8g; Sodium: 162mg; Iron: 2mg*

Blueberry Pancakes

Everyone needs a go-to pancake recipe to turn to for cozy brunches or breakfast for dinner. These are bursting with fresh blueberries and, in my mind, need nothing more than a drizzle of maple syrup to achieve perfection.

SERVES 4

Active time: 20 minutes
Total time: 20 minutes

. . . .

LOW-CARB, VEGETARIAN

½ cup almond flour

½ cup cassava flour

4 teaspoons coconut flour

1 teaspoon baking powder

½ teaspoon sea salt

4 large eggs

1 tablespoon avocado oil

1 tablespoon water

1 teaspoon vanilla extract

4 tablespoons ghee, avocado oil, or coconut oil, divided

6 ounces fresh blueberries

Maple syrup, for serving

1. **Make the batter.** Combine the almond flour, cassava flour, coconut flour, baking powder, salt, eggs, oil, water, and vanilla in a blender. Blend until smooth.

2. **Cook the pancakes.** Heat 1 tablespoon of ghee in an 8- or 10-inch nonstick pan over medium-high heat. When the oil is hot, pour about ¼ cup of batter into the pan to make a 4-inch pancake. Immediately top the pancake with several blueberries. Cook until the batter bubbles and the pancake is brown, about 2 minutes. (If the pan is smoking or the pancake browns too quickly, turn the heat to medium.) Flip the pancake and cook until the other side is browned, about 2 minutes. Transfer to a plate. Continue with the rest of the oil (as needed), batter, and blueberries, transferring the pancakes to the plate as you go.

3. **Serve.** Drizzle with maple syrup.

SIMPLE SWAP: This batter is versatile, so if you want to go savory, sub in crumbled bacon for the blueberries. For a decadent treat, try Paleo chocolate chips!

Per Serving: *Calories: 413; Fat: 31g; Protein: 12g; Total Carbs: 24g; Fiber: 3g; Sodium: 399mg; Iron: 2mg*

Baked Fruit Crepe

One of my favorite desserts is a French clafouti, which inspired this crepe (which benefits from less sugar and more protein). I love to make this on the weekends, but it comes together fast enough for a weekday breakfast, since baking the crepe instead of flipping pancakes means more hands-off time for you.

SERVES 2

Active time: 5 minutes
Total time: 25 minutes

....

5 INGREDIENTS, LOW-CARB, NUT-FREE

Olive or avocado oil spray, for greasing the pan

4 large eggs

¼ cup water

¼ cup cassava flour or arrowroot starch

1 tablespoon avocado or extra-virgin olive oil

2 scoops collagen peptides

Pinch sea salt

1½ cups fresh fruit, such as raspberries, sliced strawberries, sliced peaches, sliced plums, and/or halved cherries

Ghee and maple syrup or honey, for serving (optional)

1. **Get ready.** Preheat the oven to 400°F. Spray a 10-inch oven-safe nonstick skillet with oil and set aside.

2. **Prepare the crepe batter.** Combine the eggs, water, flour, oil, collagen, and salt in a blender. Blend until smooth.

3. **Bake the crepe.** Pour the batter into the prepared pan. Arrange the fruit on top. Bake for 20 minutes, or until set. Cut the crepe into 4 pieces. Serve hot with ghee and maple syrup or honey (if using).

COOKING HACK: I love to eat this with a couple of breakfast sausages or bacon slices. I put them on a rimmed baking sheet and pop them in the oven along with the crepe.

Per Serving *(without toppings): Calories: 252; Fat: 12g; Protein: 16g; Total Carbs: 30g; Fiber: 1g; Sodium: 158mg; Iron: 1mg*

Cherry-Berry Avocado Smoothie

Loaded with antioxidants from cherries, blueberries, and greens, this smoothie gets its dreamy creaminess (and boost in fiber) from avocado. I suggest 1 tablespoon of maple syrup as a sweetener, but you can substitute a few drops of stevia if you want to keep it lower carbohydrate. If you're interested in boosting the anti-inflammatory properties even further, add a few drops of liquid chlorophyll, available in health food stores and online.

SERVES 1

Active time: 10 minutes
Total time: 10 minutes
....
NO-COOK, NUT-FREE,
ONE-PAN, SUPER FAST

1 cup water or your favorite dairy-free milk, or more as needed

1 cup packed fresh spinach or "power greens" mix

¼ cup frozen cherries

¼ cup frozen blueberries

½ ripe avocado, pitted and peeled

1 tablespoon maple syrup or honey

1 teaspoon ground cinnamon

3 ice cubes

Pinch sea salt

2 or 3 scoops collagen peptides

1. **Make the smoothie.** Combine the water, spinach, cherries, blueberries, avocado, maple syrup, cinnamon, ice cubes, and salt in a blender. Start blending slowly, then gradually increase the speed to high and blend until the mixture is completely smooth. (If the smoothie is too thick, turn the blender off and add a bit more water; gradually increase the speed to blend it in.)

2. **Finish and serve.** Add the collagen and blend on medium for a few seconds to incorporate. Serve immediately.

SIMPLE SWAP: Substitute ½ cup of frozen spinach or kale for the fresh greens.

Per Serving: *Calories: 340; Fat: 15g; Protein: 22g; Total Carbs: 36g; Fiber: 11g; Sodium: 75mg; Iron: 2mg*

Oven-Roasted Hash Salad

Oven-roasting hash instead of cooking it on the stovetop makes it so much easier to cook perfectly. Spoon it over lemony greens to boost the nutrition even more. If you have time—hello, Sunday brunch—top the hash and greens with a poached egg.

SERVES 2

Active time: 15 minutes
Total time: 25 minutes

....

LOW-CARB, NUT-FREE, ONE-PAN

8 ounces Italian sausage, cut into ½-inch pieces

2 cups sliced red cabbage

6 button mushrooms, thinly sliced

1 small sweet potato, peeled and cut into ½-inch cubes

1 garlic clove, minced

2 scallions, white and green parts, thinly sliced

½ teaspoon dried thyme

½ teaspoon dried oregano

2 tablespoons extra-virgin olive oil

½ teaspoon sea salt

Freshly ground black pepper

2 cups arugula or baby spinach

Juice of ½ lemon

2 radishes, thinly sliced, for garnish

1. **Get ready.** Preheat the oven to 425°F. Line a rimmed baking sheet with parchment paper or aluminum foil.

2. **Roast the hash.** Scatter the sausage evenly on the prepared pan. Scatter the cabbage, mushrooms, sweet potato, garlic, and scallions over the sausage. Sprinkle with the thyme and oregano, then drizzle with the olive oil. Sprinkle with the salt and a few grinds of black pepper. Roast for 15 minutes, stir a bit, and check for doneness. Roast for another 5 to 10 minutes, or until the sausage is cooked through and the vegetables are tender-crisp.

3. **Assemble the salad.** Divide the arugula between two shallow bowls. Squeeze a bit of the lemon over the arugula. Divide the hash between the bowls, on top of the arugula. Garnish with another squeeze of lemon and the radishes. Season with salt and pepper and serve immediately.

SIMPLE SWAPS:

1. You can substitute other vegetables, such as Brussels sprouts, bok choy, asparagus, carrots, celery, cauliflower, broccoli, pea pods, and/or fennel, in any combination. For even roasting, cut the vegetables into uniform pieces.

2. Swap the sausage for slab bacon cubes, ground pork, or ground beef.

Per Serving: *Calories: 485; Fat: 34g; Protein: 24g; Total Carbs: 28g; Fiber: 7g; Sodium: 952mg; Iron: 6mg*

Easy Breakfast Tacos

Eggs and sausage scrambled together, then topped with creamy avocado, are so flavorful that you won't miss the cheese. Make 'em as spicy as you want with your favorite hot sauce, or choose chorizo for the sausage. My favorite Paleo tortillas are Siete Foods' cassava and coconut tortillas.

SERVES 4

Active time: 15 minutes
Total time: 20 minutes

5 INGREDIENTS, LOW-CARB, NUT-FREE

8 Plantain Tortillas (page 159) or store-bought Paleo tortillas

8 ounces bulk breakfast sausage

8 large eggs

1 teaspoon sea salt

Freshly ground black pepper

1 ripe avocado, pitted, peeled, and cut into 8 slices

Hot sauce, for serving

1. **Get ready.** Preheat the oven to 300°F. Wrap the tortillas in aluminum foil and place in the oven. Warm the tortillas for about 15 minutes while you prepare the filling.

2. **Cook the sausage.** Crumble the sausage into a 10-inch nonstick skillet. Fry the sausage over medium heat, breaking it up until just cooked through, about 8 minutes.

3. **Cook the eggs.** In a medium bowl, whisk the eggs with the salt and several grinds of black pepper. When the sausage is cooked through, add the eggs to the pan. Using a spatula, scramble the eggs and sausage together until the eggs are cooked to just shy of your desired consistency. (They will continue to cook as they sit in the warm pan.) Remove the pan from the heat.

4. **Assemble the tacos.** Put 2 warm tortillas on each plate. Divide the egg mixture among the tortillas. Top with the avocado slices, a sprinkle of salt, and hot sauce. Serve immediately.

Per Serving *(2 tacos, using Siete Foods' cassava and coconut tortillas): Calories: 487; Fat: 52g; Protein: 23g; Total Carbs: 30g; Fiber: 6g; Sodium: 748mg; Iron: 5mg*

Caramelized Onion and Potato Frittata

A frittata is an Italian omelet that's finished in the oven. Since it doesn't need to be folded or rolled (unlike a French omelet), it's easy to fill with big-flavor ingredients. This frittata has caramelized onions and crispy potatoes, a combination with great flavor and texture. Make this frittata for brunch or a light lunch.

SERVES 4

Active time: 15 minutes
Total time: 20 minutes

. . . .
5 INGREDIENTS, LOW-CARB, NUT-FREE, VEGETARIAN

8 large eggs

1 teaspoon sea salt

½ teaspoon dried thyme

Freshly ground black pepper

¾ cup Caramelized Onions (page 164)

2 tablespoons extra-virgin olive oil

8 ounces Yukon Gold potatoes, cut into ½-inch dice

1. **Get ready.** Arrange an oven rack 8 inches from the broiler element. Preheat the broiler.

2. **Prepare the eggs.** In a large bowl, whisk the eggs with the salt, thyme, and several grinds of black pepper. Stir in the caramelized onions. Set aside.

3. **Cook the potatoes.** Heat the oil in a 10-inch oven-safe nonstick skillet over medium-high heat. When the oil is hot, add the potatoes to the pan. Fry the potatoes, stirring frequently, until soft and browned, about 8 minutes.

4. **Cook the frittata.** Add the eggs to the pan. Cook until the bottom of the frittata starts to set, about 3 minutes. Lift the edges of the frittata and tilt the pan a bit to allow the uncooked eggs to run underneath. Continue lifting and tilting until the eggs are no longer runny. Transfer the pan to the oven and broil until the top is golden brown, about 2 minutes (keep a careful eye on it). Remove from the oven and let rest for 5 minutes. Cut the frittata into 4 wedges and serve warm.

SERVING SUGGESTION: Serve with bacon or sausage to boost the protein content of the meal.

LOVE YOUR LEFTOVERS: This frittata freezes well. Cool the wedges to room temperature, wrap in plastic wrap, and freeze in a zip-top bag. Reheat in the microwave or a warm oven.

Per Serving: Calories: 255; Fat: 16g; Protein: 14g; Total Carbs: 13g; Fiber: 2g; Sodium: 728mg; Iron: 2mg

Baked Prosciutto Egg Cups

Make the whole batch of these egg cups and stash a few in the refrigerator. They reheat nicely in the microwave and you can take them on the road. I suggest a spoonful of chimichurri for an extra flavor boost. If you're not taking them on the go, serve alongside a simple salad or fresh fruit.

SERVES 6

Active time: 15 minutes
Total time: 20 minutes

. . . .

5 INGREDIENTS, LOW-CARB,
NUT-FREE, ONE-PAN

Olive or avocado oil spray, for greasing the pan

12 slices prosciutto

12 teaspoons Chimichurri (page 160, optional)

12 large eggs

Sea salt

Freshly ground black pepper

1. **Get ready.** Preheat the oven to 425°F. Spray the cups of a 12-cup nonstick muffin tin with oil.

2. **Prepare the prosciutto cups.** Line each cup with 1 slice of prosciutto, making sure to cover the bottom and sides of the cup so the egg doesn't leak through. Add 1 teaspoon of chimichurri (if using). Crack an egg into each cup. Season with salt and black pepper.

3. **Bake the prosciutto cups.** Bake the egg cups for 10 minutes for sunny-side eggs or 13 minutes for over-medium eggs. Serve warm.

LOVE YOUR LEFTOVERS: Reheat the egg cups in a microwave for 20 seconds on high, or until the eggs are hot.

Per Serving (without chimichurri): Calories: 255; Fat: 20g; Protein: 22g; Total Carbs: 3g; Fiber: <1g; Sodium: 732mg; Iron: 3mg

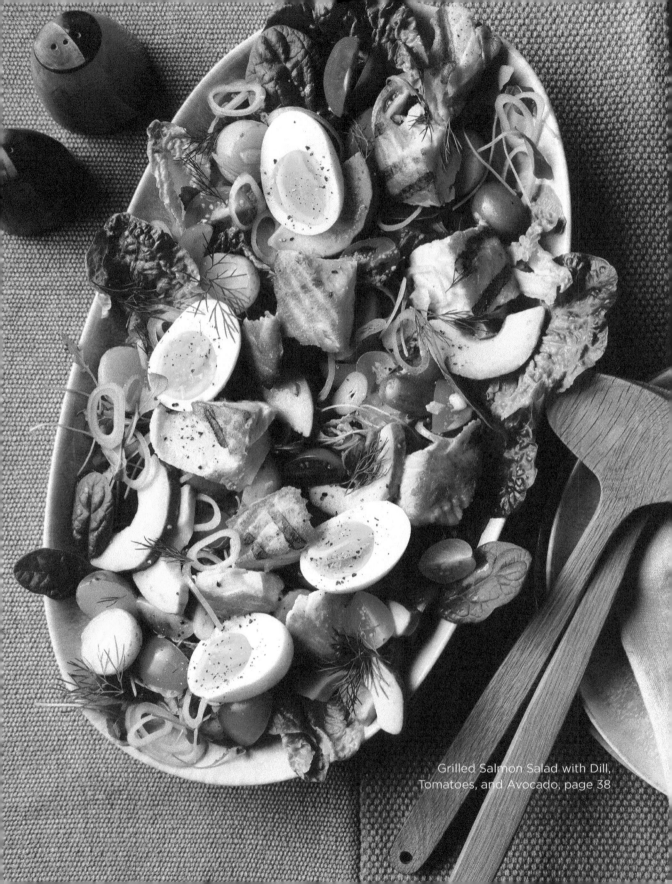

Grilled Salmon Salad with Dill, Tomatoes, and Avocado, page 38

CHAPTER THREE

Soups and Salads

Chicken, Kale, and Sweet Potato Soup

My mom had surgery a few years ago and recovered in the hospital for several days afterward. The hospital food was really awful and not very nutritious, so I created this nutrient-dense soup for her. She loved it, and it quickly became a family favorite. I make and bring this to anyone who is healing from illness, injury, or childbirth.

SERVES 4

Active time: 15 minutes
Total time: 30 minutes

LOW-CARB, NUT-FREE, ONE-PAN

3 bacon slices, chopped

1 cup finely chopped yellow onion

1 garlic clove, minced

1 teaspoon dried thyme

1 teaspoon sea salt

¼ teaspoon ground nutmeg

5 cups Rich Chicken Broth (page 158) or store-bought chicken broth

1 pound boneless, skinless chicken thighs

4 cups thinly sliced lacinato kale leaves, center ribs removed

2 cups diced, peeled sweet potato

1 tablespoon freshly squeezed lemon juice

Freshly ground black pepper

Chimichurri (page 160, optional), for garnish

1. **Cook the chicken.** In a Dutch oven or casserole with a tight-fitting lid, fry the bacon over medium-high heat until the fat is rendered and it's lightly browned, about 5 minutes. Add the onion, garlic, thyme, salt, and nutmeg and sauté, stirring occasionally, for 5 minutes. Pour in the broth and bring to a boil, then lower the heat to a simmer. Add the chicken thighs, cover, and simmer for 15 minutes.

2. **Finish the soup.** Stir in the kale and sweet potato and simmer, partially covered, for 10 minutes, or until the sweet potato is tender. Remove the chicken thighs and pull or cut them into bite-size pieces. Return the chicken to the pot. Stir in the lemon juice, then season with salt and pepper. Ladle the soup into four bowls. Add a spoonful of chimichurri (if using) and serve hot.

Per Serving *(without chimichurri): Calories: 311; Fat: 13g; Protein: 30g; Total Carbs: 17g; Fiber: 3g; Sodium: 779mg; Iron: 1mg*

Squash Soup with Sausage and Pepitas

When cooler temperatures arrive, it's time to start making all things squash. The trick for roasting squash quickly is to cut it into small enough pieces and to use high enough heat to get the browning happening quickly. Since the oven is already hot, I also roast the sausage alongside the squash.

SERVES 4

Active time: 20 minutes
Total time: 30 minutes

. . . .

LOW-CARB, NUT-FREE

1 pound precooked bratwurst or kielbasa, halved lengthwise and cut crosswise into ½-inch pieces

2 cups ½-inch diced, peeled, and seeded butternut squash

1 tablespoon extra-virgin olive oil

1 teaspoon sea salt, divided

3 cups Rich Chicken Broth (page 158) or store-bought chicken broth

½ cup canned full-fat coconut milk

¼ cup maple syrup

1 tablespoon freshly squeezed lemon juice

4 tablespoons toasted pepitas, for garnish

1. **Get ready.** Arrange two oven racks toward the middle of the oven. Preheat the oven to 425°F. Line two rimmed baking sheets with parchment paper or aluminum foil.

2. **Roast the sausage and squash.** Scatter the sausage pieces over one prepared baking sheet. Put the squash in a large bowl, drizzle with the olive oil, sprinkle with ½ teaspoon of salt, and toss to coat. Spread the squash over the second prepared baking sheet. Place both pans in the oven and roast for 15 minutes. Remove the sausage and squash from the oven.

3. **Make the soup.** Combine the broth and coconut milk in a large saucepan and bring to a simmer over medium-high heat. Add the squash and simmer for 5 minutes, or until very tender. Transfer to a blender, add the maple syrup, lemon juice, and remaining ½ teaspoon of salt, and purée until smooth. (When blending hot liquids, remove the center cap and hold a towel over the hole to allow steam to escape.) Taste the soup and add more salt, maple syrup, and/or lemon juice as needed. Ladle the soup into bowls. Divide the sausage among the bowls, top with the pepitas, and serve hot.

Continued >

SMART SHOPPING: Look for cubed squash in the produce section of your grocery store. You'll need to cut the pieces into a smaller dice, but you won't have to bother with peeling and seeding a whole squash.

COOKING HACK: Use an immersion blender to purée the soup right in the pot.

Per Serving: *Calories: 552; Fat: 41g; Protein: 19g; Total Carbs: 27g; Fiber: 2g; Sodium: 1,560mg; Iron: 2mg*

Thai Coconut Soup

Make this creamy, fragrant soup as spicy as you like by adding more (or less) sliced jalapeño—or Thai chiles, if you can find them. Look for jars of red Thai curry paste and fish sauce in the Asian section of most grocery stores. I have a feeling this soup is going to be your new go-to for cold and flu season!

SERVES 4

Active time: 20 minutes
Total time: 30 minutes

....

LOW-CARB, NUT-FREE, ONE-PAN

1 tablespoon coconut oil

½ medium yellow onion, thinly sliced

1 jalapeño, seeded (if desired) and thinly sliced

2 tablespoons minced fresh ginger

1 tablespoon red Thai curry paste

1 pound boneless, skinless chicken thighs, halved lengthwise and cut crosswise into ¼-inch-wide strips

3 cups Rich Chicken Broth (page 158) or store-bought chicken broth

1 (13.5-ounce) can full-fat coconut milk

Grated zest and juice of 1 lime

2 tablespoons maple syrup

2 tablespoons fish sauce

4 tablespoons chopped fresh cilantro, for garnish

1. **Prepare the broth.** Heat the coconut oil in a large saucepan over medium heat. When the oil is hot, add the onion and sauté until starting to soften, about 5 minutes. Add the jalapeño, ginger, curry paste, and chicken and sauté for 5 minutes. Add the broth, coconut milk, and lime zest and bring to a simmer.

2. **Simmer the soup.** Turn the heat to low, partially cover the pan, and simmer the soup for 15 minutes, or until the chicken is tender.

3. **Finish the soup.** Remove the pan from the heat. Stir in the lime juice, maple syrup, and fish sauce. Taste and add more lime juice, maple syrup, and/or fish sauce as needed. Ladle the soup into bowls, top with the cilantro, and serve hot.

Per Serving: *Calories: 398; Fat: 28g; Protein: 27g; Total Carbs: 15g; Fiber: 3g; Sodium: 1,091mg; Iron: 2mg*

Cold Melon Soup

Nothing is more refreshing on a hot day than cold melon soup. Enjoy it for lunch along with a protein-packed salad, or if you're entertaining, pour the soup into small juice glasses and serve it as an appetizer. To serve the soup without chilling it, use a ripe cantaloupe that's cold from the refrigerator. Alternatively, you can add 2 ice cubes to the blender before you blend.

SERVES 4

Active time: 10 minutes
Total time: 10 minutes

5 INGREDIENTS, LOW-CARB,
NO-COOK, NUT-FREE, ONE-PAN,
SUPER FAST, VEGETARIAN

4 heaping cups cubed ripe cantaloupe

2 tablespoons freshly squeezed
    lemon juice

1 tablespoon honey

1 tablespoon extra-virgin olive oil

½ teaspoon sea salt

Pinch cayenne pepper

1. **Make the soup.** Combine the cantaloupe, lemon juice, honey, olive oil, salt, and cayenne in a blender and blend, slowly increasing the speed, until very smooth and frothy. Taste and adjust the seasoning as needed.

2. **Serve.** Pour the soup into bowls or teacups and serve right away.

SERVING SUGGESTION: Floating bits of crispy prosciutto on top of the soup looks beautiful—and tastes delicious. Simply lay 4 pieces of prosciutto on a parchment-lined rimmed baking sheet and bake at 400°F for a few minutes until lightly browned. Cool and break into shards.

Per Serving: *Calories: 108; Fat: 4g; Protein: 2g; Total Carbs: 19g; Fiber: 2g; Sodium: 319mg; Iron: <1mg*

Gazpacho with Crispy Shrimp

Make this cold, spicy tomato soup when you have access to good garden-ripe tomatoes. You don't have to make the crispy shrimp garnish, but the pairing is so, so good. I got the idea when I ordered them together in a Palm Beach restaurant—and the two were thereafter married in my mind.

SERVES 4

Active time: 15 minutes
Total time: 15 minutes

....

LOW-CARB, NUT-FREE

FOR THE GAZPACHO

3 large garden-ripe tomatoes, cored and cut into 1-inch pieces

2 garlic cloves, coarsely chopped

1 medium cucumber, peeled, halved, seeded, and cut into 1-inch pieces

1 jalapeño, seeded (if desired) and chopped

2 cups tomato juice

½ cup coarsely chopped red onion

½ cup chopped fresh parsley

2 tablespoons red wine vinegar

2 tablespoons extra-virgin olive oil

1 teaspoon smoked paprika

1 teaspoon sea salt (or to taste, depending on how salty your tomato juice is)

Freshly ground black pepper

FOR THE SHRIMP

8 large or 12 medium shrimp, peeled and deveined

Avocado oil, for frying

1 cup tapioca starch

1 teaspoon salt

1. **Make the gazpacho.** Combine the tomatoes, garlic, cucumber, jalapeño, tomato juice, onion, parsley, vinegar, olive oil, paprika, salt, and pepper in a blender and purée until the mixture is almost smooth but still has a little texture. Taste and adjust the seasoning as needed. Chill in the refrigerator while you make the shrimp.

2. **Prepare the shrimp.** If the shrimp are wet, pat them dry a bit with paper towels. Heat a 10-inch skillet over medium-high heat. Add ½ inch of oil and heat until hot and shimmering. While the oil heats, combine the starch and salt in a large zip-top bag. Add the shrimp to the bag, seal, and toss to coat the shrimp. Fry several shrimp at a time until golden brown on both sides, 4 to 5 minutes total, transferring them to a paper towel–lined plate as you go.

3. **Serve.** Divide the gazpacho among four soup bowls. Top with crispy shrimp and serve immediately.

Per Serving: *Calories: 335; Fat: 25g; Protein: 7g; Total Carbs: 23g; Fiber: 6g; Sodium: 832mg; Iron: 2mg*

Grilled Salmon Salad with Dill, Tomatoes, and Avocado

This beautiful salad is perfect for a weeknight dinner but also special enough for guests. Set the platter in the center of the table and let everyone serve themselves. The potatoes and salmon are both slightly warm, in contrast with the cool, crisp greens. The mustardy dressing ties it all together.

SERVES 4

Active time: 20 minutes
Total time: 25 minutes
....
LOW-CARB, NUT-FREE

FOR THE DRESSING AND SALMON

¼ cup extra-virgin olive oil

3 tablespoons freshly squeezed lemon juice

2 tablespoons Dijon mustard

1 small garlic clove, minced

½ teaspoon sea salt

4 (4-ounce) salmon fillets

FOR THE SALAD

8 ounces small new potatoes

4 large eggs

3 cups greens, such as lettuce, spinach, and/or arugula

3 tablespoons chopped fresh dill

½ cup quartered cherry tomatoes

1 large shallot, thinly sliced

1 avocado, pitted, peeled, and cut into ¼-inch slices

Freshly ground black pepper

1. **Get ready.** Preheat a grill to medium-high heat.

2. **Prepare the dressing and salmon.** In a small bowl, whisk together the oil, lemon juice, mustard, garlic, and salt. Sprinkle both sides of each salmon fillet lightly with salt, then spread 1 teaspoon of dressing on one side of each fillet. Set aside.

3. **Boil the potatoes and eggs for the salad.** Fill a large saucepan with cold, salted water. Add the potatoes and bring to a boil over high heat. Turn the heat to medium, carefully add the eggs to the pan, and set a timer for 8 minutes. When the timer goes off, use tongs or a slotted spoon to transfer the eggs to a bowl of cold water. If the potatoes are tender, drain and leave them in the warm pot; if not, continue boiling for another few minutes, then drain. Set aside.

4. **Grill the salmon.** Grill the salmon fillets until just slightly underdone, 2 to 4 minutes per side, depending on the thickness (the salmon will continue cooking while it rests). Transfer to a cutting board and let rest while you assemble the salad.

5. **Assemble the salad.** Spread the greens on a large platter. Scatter the dill over the greens. Quarter the potatoes and arrange over the greens. Top with the tomatoes, shallot, and avocado. Peel and halve the eggs and arrange on top. Spoon half the remaining dressing over the salad. Break the salmon into 2-inch pieces and place on top.

Top with the remaining dressing. Finish with a light sprinkle of salt and several grinds of black pepper. Serve immediately.

COOKING HACK: If you have Chimichurri (see page 160) on hand, you can use it as a shortcut to make a dressing: In a small bowl, whisk together ⅓ cup of Chimichurri and 2 tablespoons of Dijon mustard.

Per Serving: *Calories: 483; Fat: 32g; Protein: 33g; Total Carbs: 18g; Fiber: 6g; Sodium: 582mg; Iron: 3mg*

Steak Salad with Sweet Potatoes, Avocado, and Maple Vinaigrette

Grilled steak really shines when paired with a lightly sweet vinaigrette. I chose maple syrup instead of honey because maple and sweet potatoes are one of the world's great flavor combinations; apple cider vinegar keeps the sweetness in check. If you don't have access to a grill, feel free to broil or panfry the steak.

SERVES 4

Active time: 20 minutes
Total time: 25 minutes

. . . .
NUT-FREE

FOR THE SWEET POTATOES

1 pound sweet potatoes, peeled and
  cut into ½-inch cubes

2 tablespoons extra-virgin olive oil

1 tablespoon maple syrup

½ teaspoon sea salt

FOR THE STEAK

1 (1-pound) flatiron or sirloin steak

Sea salt

FOR THE VINAIGRETTE

3 tablespoons extra-virgin olive oil

2 tablespoons maple syrup

2 tablespoons apple cider vinegar

½ teaspoon sea salt

FOR THE SALAD

4 cups torn romaine lettuce leaves

½ cup thinly sliced red onion

1 avocado, pitted, peeled, and cut into
  ¼-inch slices

Sea salt

Freshly ground black pepper

1. **Get ready.** Preheat a grill to medium-high heat. Preheat the oven to 425°F. Line a rimmed baking sheet with parchment paper or aluminum foil.

2. **Roast the sweet potatoes.** In a medium bowl, combine the sweet potatoes, oil, maple syrup, and salt and toss to evenly coat the sweet potatoes. Dump the sweet potatoes onto the prepared baking sheet, scraping any remaining oil and syrup from the bowl over the potatoes. Roast, stirring

halfway through, for 20 minutes, or until tender and lightly browned. Set aside.

3. **Grill the steak.** Meanwhile, season the steak lightly with salt. Grill for 4 to 6 minutes per side, depending on the thickness and your desired doneness. Let the steak rest on a cutting board for 5 minutes, then slice very thinly against the grain.

4. **Make the vinaigrette.** While the steak rests, combine the olive oil, maple syrup, vinegar, and salt in a small bowl and whisk. Set aside.

5. **Assemble the salad.** Divide the romaine among four plates. Add the onion and avocado. Top with the sweet potatoes and steak. Drizzle with the vinaigrette. Finish with a sprinkle of salt and a few grinds of black pepper and serve.

SIMPLE SWAP: Substitute butternut or delicata squash for the sweet potatoes.

Per Serving: *Calories: 520; Fat: 30g; Protein: 28g; Total Carbs: 37g; Fiber: 7g; Sodium: 779mg; Iron: 3mg*

Crispy Chicken and Peach Salad

Make this salad at the height of peach season and marvel at how perfectly fried chicken and peaches go together. The chicken's breading is light and comes together quickly. I suggest peppery arugula for the salad greens, but lettuce or spinach work really well, too.

SERVES 4

Active time: 25 minutes
Total time: 25 minutes

......
NUT-FREE

FOR THE DRESSING

3 tablespoons lemon juice

2 tablespoons honey

1 tablespoon extra-virgin olive oil

½ teaspoon sea salt

FOR THE SALAD

4 cups arugula

¼ cup fresh mint leaves, torn

4 radishes, very thinly sliced

2 ripe peaches or nectarines, pitted and cut into ¼-inch-thick slices

4 scallions, white and green parts, thinly sliced

Sea salt

Freshly ground black pepper

FOR THE CHICKEN

1 large egg

½ cup cassava flour

½ teaspoon sea salt

4 boneless, skinless chicken breast halves (about 1 pound), cut into ¾-inch strips

Avocado oil, for frying

1. **Make the dressing.** Whisk together the lemon juice, honey, olive oil, and salt in a small bowl until combined. Set aside.

2. **Prepare the salad.** Divide the arugula, mint, radishes, peaches, and scallions among four plates. Season with salt and pepper. Set aside.

3. **Prepare the chicken.** In a pie plate, lightly beat the egg. Combine the flour and salt in a large zip-top bag. Dip the chicken strips in the beaten egg, then put them in the bag, seal, and toss around to coat the chicken. Heat ¼ inch of oil in a 10-inch nonstick skillet over medium-high heat. When the oil is hot, fry the chicken strips, a few at a time, until nicely browned, about 3 minutes per side. Transfer to a paper towel–lined plate as you go.

4. **Assemble the salad.** When all of the chicken is cooked, slice the strips diagonally into 1-inch pieces and set atop the salads. Drizzle with the vinaigrette and serve immediately.

Per Serving: Calories: 406; Fat: 21g; Protein: 25g; Total Carbs: 31g; Fiber: 2g; Sodium: 943mg; Iron: 2mg

Shrimp Caesar Salad with Bacon-Brussels "Croutons"

I know, I know, Caesar salad is all about the cheese and croutons. And yet by making "croutons" from bacon and roasted Brussels sprouts and using avocado for the dressing, you get the feel of the salty, crunchy creaminess that a great Caesar delivers, plus a whole lot more nutrition! Shrimp and lemon go great together, and I love adding warm shrimp to Caesar salad to boost the protein.

SERVES 4

Active time: 25 minutes
Total time: 30 minutes

. . . .

LOW-CARB, NUT-FREE

FOR THE DRESSING

¼ cup freshly squeezed lemon juice

1 tablespoon fish sauce

½ ripe avocado, pitted, peeled, and mashed

3 garlic cloves, minced

½ teaspoon sea salt

½ cup extra-virgin olive oil

Freshly ground black pepper

FOR THE SALAD

2 bacon slices, cut into ½-inch pieces

2 cups thinly sliced Brussels sprouts

2 tablespoons avocado oil, divided

½ teaspoon sea salt, divided

1 pound medium or large shrimp, peeled and deveined

Freshly ground black pepper

4 cups torn romaine lettuce leaves

1. **Get ready.** Arrange an oven rack 8 inches from the broiler element and another rack toward the center of the oven. Preheat the oven to 425°F. Line a rimmed baking sheet with parchment paper and another with aluminum foil.

2. **Make the dressing.** Combine the lemon juice, fish sauce, avocado, garlic, and salt in a blender. Purée and, with the blender running, slowly drizzle in the olive oil. Taste and season with salt as needed. Add several grinds of pepper and blend again. Set aside.

3. **Roast the bacon and Brussels sprouts for the salad.** In a medium bowl, combine the bacon, Brussels sprouts, 1 tablespoon of oil, and ¼ teaspoon of salt and toss to combine. Spread evenly on the parchment-lined baking sheet (reserve the bowl) and roast for 10 minutes. Stir and roast for another 5 to 10 minutes, until browned and crisp. Remove from the oven and set aside. Turn on the broiler.

Continued >

4. **Broil the shrimp.** Combine the shrimp and remaining 1 tablespoon of oil in the reserved bowl. Sprinkle with the remaining ¼ teaspoon of salt and several grinds of pepper and toss to coat. Arrange the shrimp in an even layer on the foil-lined baking sheet. Broil the shrimp for 2 to 3 minutes, until cooked through and pink.

5. **Assemble the salad.** Divide the romaine among four plates. Top with the shrimp, then add the bacon and Brussels sprouts. Drizzle the dressing over the top. Finish with several grinds of pepper and serve immediately.

SIMPLE SWAP: You can substitute 4 mashed anchovies for the fish sauce.

Per Serving: *Calories: 406; Fat: 30g; Protein: 27g; Total Carbs: 10g; Fiber: 4g; Sodium: 857mg; Iron: 2mg*

Chopped Salad with Shrimp, Squash, and Figs

This salad is full of lovely fall flavors, namely figs and squash. If you can't find fresh figs, you can substitute your favorite apple variety, cut into ½-inch cubes. The beauty of a chopped salad is that you get all the elements of the salad in each bite, which makes it extra delicious.

SERVES 4

Active time: 25 minutes
Total time: 30 minutes

....

NUT-FREE

FOR THE DRESSING

¼ cup extra-virgin olive oil

2 tablespoons apple cider vinegar

2 tablespoons maple syrup

1 shallot, minced

1 teaspoon sea salt

FOR THE SALAD

1 to 2 pounds delicata squash, halved lengthwise, seeded, and cut into ½-inch slices

1 tablespoon extra-virgin olive oil

Sea salt

1 pound medium or large shrimp, peeled and deveined

4 bacon slices, cut into ½-inch pieces

4 cups torn romaine lettuce leaves

8 ripe figs, trimmed and quartered

4 radishes, cut into ½-inch cubes

4 tablespoons sliced scallions, white and green parts

Freshly ground black pepper

1. **Get ready.** Preheat the oven to 400°F. Line a rimmed baking sheet with parchment paper or aluminum foil.

2. **Make the dressing.** In a small bowl, whisk together the oil, vinegar, maple syrup, shallot, and salt. Taste and adjust the seasoning as needed and set aside.

3. **Roast the squash for the salad.** In a medium bowl, toss the squash with the olive oil, sprinkle with salt, and toss to coat. Spread the squash on the prepared baking sheet and roast for 10 minutes. Turn the squash over and roast for another 10 minutes, until tender and browning at the edges. Halve the squash slices right on the baking sheet. Set aside.

4. **Cook the bacon and shrimp.** In a medium bowl, toss the shrimp with 2 tablespoons of the dressing and a generous pinch of salt; set aside. In a large skillet, fry the bacon over medium heat, stirring occasionally, until crisp, about 5 minutes. Using a

Continued >

slotted spoon, transfer the bacon to a paper towel–lined plate to drain. Pour off all but 1 tablespoon of bacon drippings from the pan (reserve for another use). Return the pan to the heat and add the shrimp. Cook for 3 to 4 minutes per side, until just cooked through. Remove the pan from the heat. Halve each shrimp right in the pan.

5. **Assemble the salad.** Divide the romaine among four plates and drizzle with a bit of the dressing. Divide the figs, radishes, and scallions among the plates. Top with the squash, bacon, and shrimp. Drizzle with a bit more dressing and top with a sprinkle of salt and a few grinds of pepper. Serve while the shrimp and squash are still warm.

Per Serving: *Calories: 453; Fat: 25g; Protein: 21g; Total Carbs: 38g; Fiber: 6g; Sodium: 763mg; Iron: 2mg*

Classic Broccoli Salad

This salad goes by various names, including sunshine salad. My version includes cashews and a dressing much lower in sugar than a traditional one. This is the rare salad that actually improves with sitting, so it's fantastic for taking to a party (you can double or triple the recipe easily). It stands alone, but I also love it paired with grilled barbecue chicken—pure summer.

SERVES 4

Active time: 25 minutes
Total time: 30 minutes

. . . .
LOW-CARB

½ cup Mayonnaise (page 166) or store-bought Paleo mayonnaise

2 tablespoons apple cider vinegar

2 tablespoons coconut sugar

8 ounces thick-sliced bacon, cut into ¾-inch pieces

12 ounces (1-inch) broccoli florets

½ cup salted toasted cashews

¼ medium red onion, finely chopped

¼ cup dried cherries

1. **Make the dressing.** In a small bowl, stir together the mayonnaise, vinegar, and sugar (the sugar will dissolve while you cook the bacon). Set aside.

2. **Cook the bacon.** Heat a 12-inch skillet over medium heat. Add the bacon and fry, stirring frequently, until evenly browned and crisp, about 7 minutes. Using a slotted spoon, transfer the bacon to a paper towel–lined plate. (Save the bacon drippings for another use.)

3. **Assemble the salad.** Combine the broccoli, cashews, onion, cherries, and bacon in a large bowl. Stir the dressing, then pour half of it over the salad. Stir to coat the salad with dressing. Taste and add more dressing as needed. (You might not use it all; cover and refrigerate leftover dressing and use for other salads.) Serve immediately.

SIMPLE SWAP: To make this dish vegetarian, omit the bacon and double the amount of cashews.

Per Serving: *Calories: 407; Fat: 36g; Protein: 10g; Total Carbs: 15g; Fiber: <1g; Sodium: 307mg; Iron: 2mg*

Salade Niçoise

Salade Niçoise is the perfect way to elevate a humble can of tuna. Choose tuna packed in olive oil for the most tender fish. I cook the eggs just shy of hardboiled, with a slightly jammy yolk, but if you prefer hardboiled, boil for 10 minutes instead of 8.

SERVES 4

Active time: 20 minutes
Total time: 25 minutes

LOW-CARB, NUT-FREE

FOR THE DRESSING

1 garlic clove, minced

⅓ cup extra-virgin olive oil

2 tablespoons red wine vinegar

1 tablespoon Dijon mustard

1 teaspoon dried thyme

½ teaspoon sea salt

Freshly ground black pepper

FOR THE SALAD

8 ounces 1-inch new potatoes (if larger, halved)

4 large eggs

8 ounces green beans, trimmed

4 cups torn romaine lettuce leaves

1 cup halved cherry tomatoes

⅓ cup thinly sliced red onion

⅓ cup Niçoise or kalamata olives

2 (5-ounce) cans tuna in olive oil, drained

Sea salt

Freshly ground black pepper

1. **Make the dressing.** In a small bowl, whisk together the garlic, olive oil, vinegar, mustard, thyme, salt, and pepper. Set aside.

2. **Boil the potatoes, green beans, and eggs.** Fill a large pot with cold, salted water, add the potatoes, and bring to a boil over high heat. Turn the heat to medium-high and carefully add the eggs to the pan. Set a timer for 4 minutes. When the timer goes off, add the green beans to the pot and again set the timer for 4 minutes. When the timer goes off a second time, use tongs or a slotted spoon to transfer the eggs to a bowl of cold water. Drain the potatoes and green beans. Set aside.

3. **Assemble the salad.** Divide the lettuce among four plates. Drizzle dressing over the lettuce. Top each plate with the tomatoes, onion, olives, potatoes, and green beans. Top with tuna. Peel the eggs, halve, and add to the plates. Top the salads with more dressing, salt, and a few grinds of pepper. Serve immediately.

Per Serving: Calories: 475; Fat: 30g; Protein: 30g; Total Carbs: 22g; Fiber: 4g; Sodium: 794mg; Iron: 4mg

Healing Green Broth

I created this addictive soup a few years ago and published it on my blog, Fresh Tart. Within a month or two, it had taken on a life of its own. It's very energizing and satisfying and just makes people feel good. Making it in a high-powered blender does make a big difference in achieving a smooth, creamy consistency. Use whatever herbs you like or have on hand.

MAKES 1 SERVING

Active time: 10 minutes
Total time: 10 minutes

....

LOW-CARB, NUT-FREE

1 cup Rich Chicken Broth (page 158) or store-bought chicken broth

1 cup watercress or arugula leaves

2 tablespoons chopped fresh tarragon

2 tablespoons chopped fresh chervil

2 tablespoons chopped fresh chives

1 tablespoon freshly squeezed lemon juice

1 tablespoon ghee, extra-virgin olive, or avocado oil

1 tablespoon MCT (medium-chain triglycerides) oil (optional)

1 tablespoon collagen peptides (optional)

Sea salt

1. **Make the broth.** In a small saucepan, bring the chicken broth to a simmer over high heat. Meanwhile, combine the watercress, tarragon, chervil, chives, lemon juice, ghee, MCT oil (if using), and collagen (if using) in a high-powered blender. Carefully pour the hot chicken broth into the blender and blend on high speed until pale green and frothy. (When blending hot liquids, remove the center cap and hold a towel over the hole to allow steam to escape.)

2. **Serve.** Season with salt and serve immediately.

Per Serving *(without MCT oil or collagen): Calories: 297; Fat: 28g; Protein: 10g; Total Carbs: 5g; Fiber: 1g; Sodium: 147mg; Iron: 2mg*

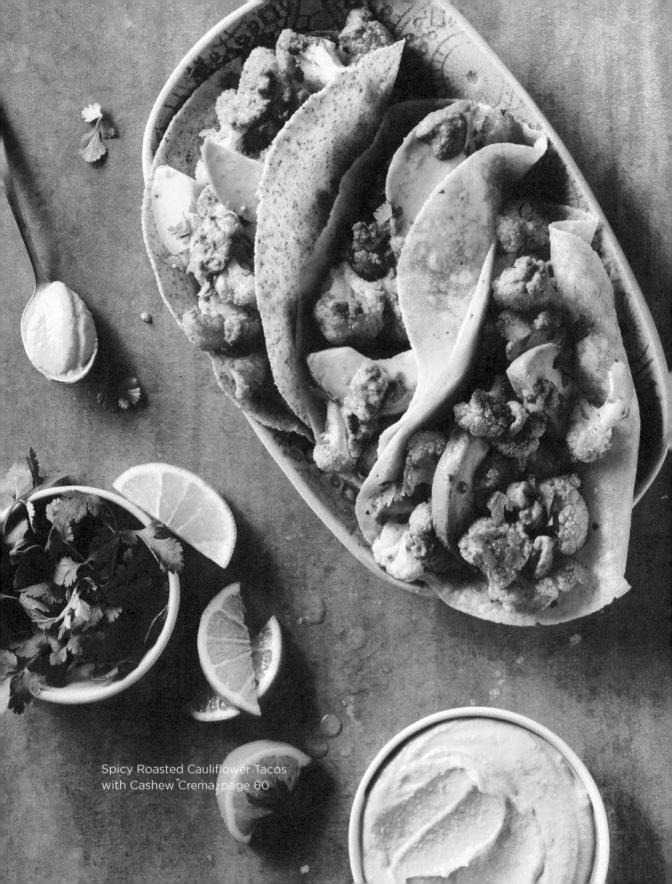

Spicy Roasted Cauliflower Tacos
with Cashew Crema, page 60

Vegetables

Bibimbap Bowl

Bibimbap is a flavor-bomb Korean rice bowl dish, topped with an assortment of cooked and raw vegetables, pickles, and a fried egg. To keep this recipe fast, I suggest using kimchi, which is available in the refrigerator section of most supermarkets, with other chilled pickles. As a fermented food, it's loaded with probiotics and keeps well in the refrigerator.

SERVES 4

Active time: 25 minutes
Total time: 30 minutes

LOW-CARB, NUT-FREE, VEGETARIAN

FOR THE CAULIFLOWER

4 cups frozen cauliflower rice (or grind 4 cups cauliflower florets in a food processor)

1 tablespoon avocado oil

1 teaspoon sea salt

FOR THE SAUCE

2 tablespoons toasted sesame oil

2 tablespoons coconut aminos

2 tablespoons maple syrup

1 tablespoon apple cider vinegar

1 tablespoon sriracha

FOR THE TOPPINGS

3 tablespoons ghee or avocado oil, divided

6 ounces button mushrooms, sliced

Sea salt

6 cups baby spinach

1 garlic clove, thinly sliced

½ cup kimchi

4 scallions, green parts only, thinly sliced, for garnish

2 tablespoons sesame seeds, for garnish

FOR THE EGGS

1 tablespoon avocado oil, divided

8 large eggs

Sea salt

1. **Get ready.** Preheat the oven to 425°F and line a rimmed baking sheet with parchment paper or aluminum foil.

2. **Roast the cauliflower.** In a large bowl, combine the cauliflower rice, oil, and salt. Toss to coat. Spread the cauliflower on the prepared baking sheet and roast for 10 minutes. Stir and roast for another 5 to 10 minutes, until browned at the edges.

3. **Make the sauce.** Meanwhile, in a small bowl, stir together the sesame oil, coconut aminos, maple syrup, vinegar, and sriracha and set aside.

4. **Make the toppings.** Heat 2 tablespoons of ghee in a 10-inch

nonstick pan over medium heat. When the ghee is hot, add the mushrooms and a generous pinch of salt. Sauté until the mushrooms are lightly browned, about 7 minutes, then transfer to a bowl. Return the pan to the heat and add the remaining 1 tablespoon of ghee. When the ghee is hot, add the spinach and a generous pinch of salt. Sauté until the spinach is wilted, about 3 minutes. Add the garlic and sauté for 1 minute more. Transfer the spinach and garlic to the bowl with the mushrooms.

5. **Assemble the bibimbap.** Divide the cauliflower among four shallow bowls. Divide the mushrooms and spinach among the bowls. Add a spoonful of kimchi to each bowl.

6. **Fry the eggs and finish the dish.** Heat ½ tablespoon of oil in the pan over medium-high heat. When the oil is hot, add 4 eggs and a pinch of salt and fry to your desired doneness. Transfer the eggs to two of the bowls. Repeat the process with the remaining ½ tablespoon of oil and 4 eggs. Drizzle the sauce over each bowl. Sprinkle with scallions and sesame seeds. To eat the bowls, break into the eggs and mix everything together a bit.

Per Serving: *Calories: 439; Fat: 34g; Protein: 19g; Total Carbs: 19g; Fiber: 5g; Sodium: 1,356mg; Iron: 5mg*

Thai Omelets in Coconut Curry Broth

This dish is inspired by a stand at my favorite farmers' market. The chef serves quick-cooked Thai dishes on Sundays, and this dish in particular really hits the spot. When I created this recipe, I ran it by him and he gave it a thumbs-up!

SERVES 4

Active time: 20 minutes
Total time: 20 minutes

....

LOW-CARB, NUT-FREE, VEGETARIAN

FOR THE BROTH

1 (13.5-ounce) can full-fat coconut milk

2 tablespoons Thai green curry paste

1 cup thinly sliced cabbage

½ cup vegetable broth

2 tablespoons coconut aminos

2 tablespoons maple syrup

Grated zest and juice of ½ lime

FOR THE OMELETS

8 large eggs

¼ cup chopped fresh basil

¼ cup chopped fresh cilantro

4 teaspoons coconut aminos

4 teaspoons avocado oil, divided

4 tablespoons thinly sliced scallions, green parts only, for garnish

Sriracha, for garnish (optional)

1. **Make the broth.** Spoon some of the fat from the top of the can of coconut milk into a medium saucepan set over medium heat. When the fat is hot, stir in the curry paste and cabbage and fry for 5 minutes. Stir in the rest of the coconut milk, the broth, coconut aminos, and maple syrup. Simmer until the cabbage is tender, about 5 minutes. Mix in the lime zest and juice. Set aside and keep warm.

2. **Make the omelets and finish the dish.** In a medium bowl, beat the eggs with the basil, cilantro, and coconut aminos. Heat 1 teaspoon of oil in a 10-inch non-stick skillet over medium-high heat. When the oil is very hot, add ½ cup of the egg mixture to the pan. Swirl the egg around in the pan, and when the edges start to brown—which will be quickly—use a spatula to fold the omelet in half and then in half again. Cook for a few more minutes, then transfer to a bowl. Ladle one-quarter of the broth over the top. Repeat the process with the remaining oil, egg mixture, and broth. Sprinkle each bowl with the scallions and top with sriracha (if using). Serve immediately.

SERVING SUGGESTION: Add a serving of hot cauliflower rice to each bowl.

Per Serving *(without sriracha): Calories: 427; Fat: 35g; Protein: 15g; Total Carbs: 18g; Fiber: 5g; Sodium: 352mg; Iron: 7mg*

Veggie Pizza

The trick to working with a dough this sticky is to roll it out between parchment paper and a sheet of plastic wrap. You bake the dough right on top of the parchment paper for quick, no-fuss handling. (Or you can use a store-bought Paleo crust.) The combination of mushrooms, tomatoes, red onion, and olives delivers a big flavor punch.

SERVES 4

Active time: 30 minutes
Total time: 30 minutes

LOW-CARB, VEGETARIAN

FOR THE PIZZA CRUST

¾ cup arrowroot starch

½ cup almond flour

5 tablespoons coconut flour

1 teaspoon dried oregano

1 teaspoon sea salt

⅓ cup water

⅓ cup extra-virgin olive oil

1 tablespoon apple cider vinegar

1 large egg

FOR THE TOPPINGS

2 tablespoons extra-virgin olive oil

2 cups sliced button mushrooms

Sea salt

1 garlic clove, minced

1 cup Cashew Cheese
  (page 163, optional)

½ cup chopped tomatoes

½ cup thinly sliced red onion

½ cup sliced green or black olives

Freshly ground black pepper

2 tablespoons Chimichurri (page 160)
  or ¼ cup chopped fresh basil

1. **Get ready.** Preheat the oven to 450°F.

2. **Prepare the dough.** Combine the arrowroot, almond flour, coconut flour, oregano, and salt in a food processor and pulse a couple of times. Add the water, oil, vinegar, and egg and pulse just until the dough comes together in a ball. Be careful not to overprocess.

3. **Make the crust.** Lay out a 14-inch piece of parchment paper. Place the dough ball on the parchment paper and flatten it a bit with your hands. Top the dough ball with a 14-inch piece of plastic wrap. With a rolling pin, roll the dough into a 12-inch circle. Peel away the plastic wrap. With a pizza peel, or using an inverted baking sheet, transfer the crust—including the parchment paper—to the oven rack. Bake for 10 minutes.

Continued >

4. **Sauté the mushrooms for the toppings.** While the crust bakes, heat the oil in a 10-inch nonstick skillet over medium-high heat. When the oil is hot, add the mushrooms and a generous pinch of salt. Sauté until the mushrooms are browning, about 7 minutes. Stir in the garlic and set aside.

5. **Top and finish the pizza.** When the crust has baked for 10 minutes, use the pizza peel or baking sheet to remove the crust (and parchment paper) from the oven. Cover the crust with the cashew cheese (if using), cooked mushrooms, tomatoes, onion, olives, and a sprinkle of salt. Return the pizza (and parchment paper) to the oven and bake for another 10 minutes. Transfer the pizza to a cutting board and cut into wedges. Grind pepper on top, drizzle with a bit of chimichurri (if using), and serve.

Per Serving (*without cashew cheese or chimichurri*)*: Calories: 461; Fat: 38g; Protein: 6g; Total Carbs: 28g; Fiber: 4g; Sodium: 762mg; Iron: 1mg*

Cold Sesame Noodle Salad

If you've had a habit of take-out sesame noodles, I think this recipe will cure you of it. It comes together so quickly, from mostly pantry ingredients, and immediately delivers the creamy-salty-nutty-sweet deliciousness of cold sesame noodles. I've added cabbage to boost the nutrition.

SERVES 4

Active time: 15 minutes
Total time: 20 minutes

VEGAN

6 ounces sweet potato starch noodles (aka japchae or "glass" noodles)

⅓ cup crunchy almond butter or sunflower seed butter

¼ cup coconut aminos

3 tablespoons toasted sesame oil

3 tablespoons apple cider vinegar

1 teaspoon sriracha

2 tablespoons minced red onion

3 garlic cloves, minced

2 teaspoons minced fresh ginger

2 cups thinly sliced green cabbage

½ medium cucumber, peeled, seeded, and cut into matchsticks

4 scallions, white and green parts, cut into 4-inch pieces

2 tablespoons sesame seeds, for garnish

1. **Boil the noodles.** Fill a large pot with cold, salted water and bring to a boil over high heat. Add the noodles and cook according to the package directions; drain and rinse with cool water. If the noodles are very long, use scissors to trim them to 8 inches.

2. **Make the sauce.** Stir together the almond butter, coconut aminos, sesame oil, vinegar, sriracha, onion, garlic, and ginger. If necessary, add warm water, 1 teaspoon at a time, until the sauce is the consistency of cream.

3. **Assemble the salad.** In a large bowl, toss the cabbage, cucumber, and scallions. If the noodles have gotten sticky, rinse them in cold water again and drain thoroughly. Add the noodles to the bowl. Top with the sauce and toss to coat. Sprinkle with the sesame seeds and serve.

Per Serving: Calories: 410; Fat: 18g; Protein: 6g; Total Carbs: 59g; Fiber: 4g; Sodium: 476mg; Iron: 3mg

Zucchini Noodle Pad Thai

I'll never forget the first time I had pad thai in a restaurant. I couldn't imagine how there were so many wonderful flavors in one dish. It was my introduction to the hallmark balance of salty, sweet, tangy, and savory that makes Thai food so incredibly delicious. Instead of the usual peanuts, I use toasted walnuts in this dish, but you could also use almonds or pecans if you prefer.

SERVES 4

Active time: 15 minutes
Total time: 20 minutes

LOW-CARB, VEGETARIAN

FOR THE SAUCE

¼ cup apple cider vinegar

¼ cup coconut aminos

¼ cup tomato paste

2 tablespoons maple syrup

2 to 3 teaspoons sriracha

FOR THE NOODLES

3 tablespoons avocado oil, divided

4 medium zucchini, cut into noodles with a spiralizer or julienne peeler

6 ounces button mushrooms, sliced

4 scallions, thinly sliced, white and green parts

3 garlic cloves, minced

1 red bell pepper, seeded and thinly sliced

3 large eggs, lightly beaten

⅔ cup chopped walnuts, toasted

½ cup chopped fresh cilantro

1 lime, cut into 4 wedges, for serving

1. **Make the sauce.** In a small bowl, combine the vinegar, coconut aminos, tomato paste, maple syrup, and sriracha. Set aside.

2. **Cook the noodles.** Heat 1 tablespoon of oil in a 12-inch nonstick skillet over medium heat. When the oil is hot, add the zucchini noodles. Sauté until tender-crisp, about 3 minutes. Transfer the noodles to a bowl. Heat the remaining 2 tablespoons of oil in the same skillet, then add the mushrooms, scallions, garlic, and bell pepper. Sauté until the bell pepper is tender-crisp and the mushrooms are browning, about 7 minutes. Pour the eggs into the pan and scramble into the vegetables.

3. **Finish the dish.** Using tongs, lift the zucchini noodles from the bowl, leaving behind any excess liquid at the bottom of the bowl, and add them to the pan. Stir in the sauce and cook until hot, about 2 minutes. Remove the pan from the heat. Stir in the walnuts and cilantro. Serve with the lime wedges.

SMART SHOPPING: Zucchini noodles ("zoodles") can be found in the produce section of many grocery stores.

SERVING SUGGESTION: To add protein to this pad thai, toss in 1 pound of broiled, peeled, and deveined shrimp as you finish the dish. To broil, add the shrimp and 1 tablespoon of avocado oil to a medium bowl. Sprinkle with ½ teaspoon of sea salt and several grinds of black pepper and toss to coat. Arrange the shrimp in an even layer on a foil-lined baking sheet. Broil for 2 to 3 minutes, or until the shrimp are cooked through and pink.

Per Serving: Calories: 343; Fat: 27g; Protein: 11g; Total Carbs: 17g; Fiber: 3g; Sodium: 569mg; Iron: 3mg

Spicy Roasted Cauliflower Tacos with Cashew Crema

Cauliflower and cashews are the chameleons of Paleo cooking. Here they're paired together in tacos, with spicy roasted cauliflower as the filling and cashews blended into a creamy sauce. Make sure to load these tacos up with cilantro and avocado to really fill out the meal. My favorite Paleo tortillas are Siete Foods, cassava and coconut tortillas.

SERVES 4

Active time: 20 minutes
Total time: 25 minutes
....
VEGAN

FOR THE CAULIFLOWER AND TORTILLAS

8 cups (1-inch) cauliflower florets

3 tablespoons avocado oil

4 teaspoons ground cumin

1 to 2 teaspoons chipotle powder

1 teaspoon sea salt

8 Plantain Tortillas (page 159) or
   store-bought Paleo tortillas

FOR THE CASHEW CREMA

1 cup raw or toasted cashews

½ cup water

1 tablespoon freshly squeezed lime juice

1 canned chipotle pepper (add a bit of
   the adobo sauce for more heat)

½ teaspoon sea salt

FOR SERVING

1 avocado, pitted, peeled, and cut into
   8 slices

¼ cup chopped fresh cilantro

1 lime, cut into 4 wedges

1. **Get ready.** Preheat the oven to 425°F. Line a rimmed baking sheet with parchment paper or aluminum foil.

2. **Prepare the cauliflower and tortillas.** In a large bowl, toss the cauliflower with the oil, cumin, chipotle powder, and salt. Spread the cauliflower on the prepared baking sheet and roast for 10 minutes. Turn the cauliflower over and roast for another 10 minutes, or until nicely browned in spots. During the last 5 minutes of roasting, wrap the tortillas in aluminum foil and add them to the oven. When done, remove both from oven and set aside.

3. **Prepare the cashew crema.** Meanwhile, combine the cashews, water, lime juice, chipotle, and salt in a blender and blend on high until smooth and creamy. Taste and add more salt as needed. Transfer to a small bowl.

4. **Serve the tacos.** Put 2 warm tortillas on each plate. Divide the cauliflower filling among the tortillas. Add the

avocado and cilantro and a squeeze of lime. Top with the cashew crema and serve.

SERVING SUGGESTION: If you have some Chimichurri (see page 160) on hand, it is terrific drizzled on these tacos.

Per Serving *(2 tacos made with Siete Foods' coconut and cassava tortillas): Calories: 496; Fat: 32g; Protein: 11g; Total Carbs: 51g; Fiber: 12g; Sodium: 977mg; Iron: 4mg*

Roasted Cauliflower "Couscous"

The beauty of this recipe is in the throw-togetherness of it. None of the measurements need to be exact. I've included a base recipe with suggestions for add-ins, but feel free to stir in whatever you like and adapt it to whatever vegetables and fruits are in season. Although the dish stands alone, it also makes a great side.

SERVES 4

Active time: 15 minutes
Total time: 25 minutes

LOW-CARB, VEGAN

1 large head cauliflower, cut into florets

2 tablespoons olive or avocado oil

½ teaspoon sea salt

½ cup dried cranberries, raisins, or dried cherries

½ cup sliced scallions, white and green parts

½ cup finely chopped fresh parsley

½ cup chopped kalamata olives

Grated zest of 1 lemon, plus 1 tablespoon freshly squeezed lemon juice

½ cup sliced vegetables, such as radishes, cucumber, arugula, spinach, and/or cherry tomatoes (optional)

½ cup roasted nuts and/or seeds, such as cashews, pepitas, and/or pine nuts (optional)

Sea salt

1. **Get ready.** Arrange two racks in the middle of the oven. Preheat the oven to 425°F. Line two rimmed baking sheets with parchment paper or aluminum foil.

2. **Prepare the cauliflower.** Put half the cauliflower in a food processor. Add 1 tablespoon of olive oil and ¼ teaspoon of salt and process until the cauliflower is the texture of couscous. Spread the cauliflower evenly on one prepared baking sheet. Repeat the process with the remaining cauliflower, olive oil, and salt and spread on the other prepared baking sheet.

3. **Roast the cauliflower.** Put both baking sheets in the oven and roast for 10 minutes. Stir the cauliflower and swap the sheets when you return them to the oven. Bake for 5 to 10 minutes more, until the cauliflower is just browning at the edges of the pan.

4. **Finish the dish.** Scrape the cauliflower into a large bowl and add the cranberries, scallions, parsley, olives, lemon zest, and lemon juice. Stir in the vegetables (if using) and nuts (if using). Season with salt and serve warm.

Per Serving *(without vegetable or nut add-ins): Calories: 188; Fat: 10g; Protein: 5g; Total Carbs: 26g; Fiber: 6g; Sodium: 193mg; Iron: 2mg*

Ginger Fried "Rice" with Fried Eggs

Don't let the limited number of ingredients fool you—this dish packs a ton of flavor. This recipe is inspired by the great chef Jean-Georges Vongerichten, who shared a ginger fried rice recipe years ago. I've adapted his recipe over time, using cauliflower "rice," healthier oil, scallions instead of leeks, and coconut aminos instead of soy sauce. But his idea for crispy ginger and garlic remains intact.

SERVES 4

Active time: 15 minutes
Total time: 25 minutes
....
LOW-CARB, NUT-FREE, VEGETARIAN

FOR THE CAULIFLOWER

4 cups frozen cauliflower rice (or grind
    4 cups cauliflower florets in a
    food processor)

2 tablespoons avocado oil, divided

1 teaspoon sea salt

¼ cup finely chopped fresh ginger

4 garlic cloves, finely chopped

4 scallions, white and green
    parts, chopped

FOR THE EGGS

1 tablespoon avocado oil

8 large eggs

¼ teaspoon sea salt

FOR THE GARNISH

4 teaspoons toasted sesame oil

4 teaspoons coconut aminos

Sesame seeds (optional)

1. **Get ready.** Preheat the oven to 425°F. Line a rimmed baking sheet with parchment paper or aluminum foil.

2. **Roast the cauliflower.** In a large bowl, combine the cauliflower, 1 tablespoon of oil, and the salt. Toss to coat. Spread the cauliflower on the prepared baking sheet and roast for 10 minutes. Stir the cauliflower, then roast for another 5 to 10 minutes, until browned at the edges.

3. **Fry the cauliflower rice.** Heat the remaining 1 tablespoon of oil in a 12-inch nonstick skillet over medium heat. When the oil is hot, add the ginger and garlic and stir-fry until brown and crispy, about 5 minutes. Using a slotted spoon, transfer the ginger and garlic to a plate, leaving the oil in the pan. Add the scallions to the pan and stir-fry for 1 minute, until wilted. Add the cauliflower to the pan and stir to heat and combine. Divide the cauliflower rice among four shallow bowls.

Continued >

4. **Make the eggs.** Wipe out the pan with a paper towel. Heat ½ tablespoon of oil in the pan over medium heat. When the oil is hot, add 4 eggs and a pinch of salt and fry to the desired doneness. Transfer the eggs to two of the bowls. Repeat the process with the remaining ½ tablespoon of oil and 4 eggs.

5. **Finish the dish and serve.** Drizzle 1 teaspoon each of sesame oil and coconut aminos over the eggs and cauliflower. Divide the crispy garlic and ginger over each dish. Sprinkle with sesame seeds (if using) and serve immediately.

Per Serving (*without sesame seeds*): *Calories: 290; Fat: 21g; Protein: 16g; Total Carbs: 10g; Fiber: 3g; Sodium: 903mg; Iron: 2mg*

Hash Brown Skillet Dinner

This quick, easy, and satisfying dinner requires very little chopping. A marriage between breakfast tacos and a hash, there's something for everyone here, from crispy potatoes to creamy avocado to spicy salsa. If you prefer, you can fry the eggs instead of scrambling them.

SERVES 4

Active time: 15 minutes
Total time: 25 minutes

....

LOW-CARB, NUT-FREE, VEGETARIAN

- 2 green bell peppers, seeded and cut into ½-inch strips
- 1 medium red onion, cut into ½-inch slices
- 4 tablespoons avocado oil, divided
- 1½ teaspoons sea salt, plus more as needed, divided
- 4 cups frozen hash browns
- 8 large eggs
- 1 avocado, pitted, peeled, and cut into 8 slices, for garnish
- ¼ cup red or green salsa, for garnish

1. **Get ready.** Preheat the oven to 425°F. Line a rimmed baking sheet with parchment paper or aluminum foil.

2. **Roast the vegetables.** In a large bowl, toss together the bell peppers, onion, and 1 tablespoon of oil. Season with salt. Spread the vegetables onto the prepared baking sheet and roast for 10 minutes. Toss the vegetables and roast for another 5 to 10 minutes, until browned in spots.

3. **Make the hash browns.** Meanwhile, heat 2 tablespoons of oil in a 10-inch nonstick pan over medium heat. When the oil is hot, add the hash browns to the pan. Sprinkle with ½ teaspoon of salt and cook, without disturbing, until the hash browns are brown and crispy on the bottom, about 10 minutes. Turn the hash browns over and fry on the second side until crispy, another 10 minutes. Divide the hash browns among four plates and season with salt.

4. **Scramble the eggs.** Return the pan to medium heat and add the remaining 1 tablespoon of oil. Lightly beat the eggs with the remaining 1 teaspoon of salt. Scramble the eggs to your desired doneness and spoon over the hash browns. Arrange the roasted vegetables over the eggs and top with the avocado slices and a spoonful of salsa. Serve hot.

Per Serving: *Calories: 454; Fat: 31g; Protein: 16g; Total Carbs: 28g; Fiber: 6g; Sodium: 575mg; Iron: 3mg*

Veggie Lo Mein

I really missed noodle dishes like this when I first adopted a Paleo style of eating. Discovering sweet potato starch noodles has been a game changer for me, which is why they show up a few times in this book. They're perfect for stir-frying because they hold their chewiness and don't fall apart. You can find them at Asian grocery stores or purchase them online.

SERVES 4

Active time: 15 minutes
Total time: 25 minutes

....

NUT-FREE, VEGAN

FOR THE SAUCE

2 tablespoons coconut aminos

1 tablespoon maple syrup

1 tablespoon toasted sesame oil

1 tablespoon apple cider vinegar

2 garlic cloves, minced

2 teaspoons ground ginger

FOR THE LO MEIN

6 ounces sweet potato starch noodles (aka japchae or "glass" noodles)

2 tablespoons avocado oil, plus more as needed

2 medium carrots, peeled and thinly sliced

6 ounces mushrooms, thinly sliced

3 cups thinly sliced lacinato kale

8 scallions, green parts only, cut into ¼-inch-thick slices

1. **Make the sauce.** In a small bowl, whisk together the coconut aminos, maple syrup, sesame oil, vinegar, garlic, and ginger. Set aside.

2. **Boil the noodles for the lo mein.** Fill a large pot with cold, salted water and bring to a boil over high heat. Add the noodles and cook according to the package directions; drain and rinse with cool water. If the noodles are very long, use scissors to trim them to 8 inches.

3. **Finish the dish.** Heat the oil in a wok or 12-inch nonstick skillet over medium-high heat until shimmering, about 1 minute. Add the carrots, mushrooms, and kale and stir-fry until wilted, about 8 minutes. If the noodles have gotten sticky, rinse them in cold water again and drain thoroughly. Add the noodles, scallions, and sauce. Stir-fry until the sauce cooks down, 2 to 3 minutes. Serve immediately.

SIMPLE SWAP: Substitute 2 cups of broccoli florets or sugar snap peas for the kale.

Per Serving: Calories: 286; Fat: 11g; Protein: 3g; Total Carbs: 46g; Fiber: 2g; Sodium: 269mg; Iron: 2mg

Zucchini Fritter Bowls with Dill Yogurt Sauce

Baking these fritters instead of frying saves time and a mess on the stovetop. It's important to squeeze as much liquid from the zucchini as possible, so put a little elbow grease into it. I adore savory pancakes—they make a comforting dinner or a fun twist on brunch—and in my mind, fritters are a version of a savory pancake.

SERVES 4

Active time: 20 minutes
Total time: 25 minutes

. . . .

LOW-CARB, VEGETARIAN

FOR THE ZUCCHINI FRITTERS

Olive or avocado oil spray, for greasing the pan

1 pound zucchini

½ cup finely chopped yellow onion

1 cup almond flour

1 tablespoon coconut flour

1 teaspoon ground cumin

1 teaspoon sea salt

2 large eggs, beaten

FOR THE SAUCE

1 cup plain coconut yogurt

¼ cup chopped fresh dill

1 garlic clove, chopped

½ teaspoon sea salt

Freshly ground black pepper

FOR THE BOWLS

4 cups baby spinach

1. **Get ready.** Preheat the oven to 425°F. Line a rimmed baking sheet with parchment paper or aluminum foil. Generously spray the parchment paper with oil.

2. **Prepare the fritters.** Using a box grater or the grater attachment on a food processor, grate the zucchini. Transfer the zucchini to a large dish towel. Standing over the sink, roll up the towel and twist it to squeeze as much moisture out of the zucchini as possible. Put the zucchini in a large mixing bowl and add the onion, almond flour, coconut flour, cumin, salt, and eggs. Stir to combine.

3. **Bake the fritters.** Using a spoon or ice cream scoop, form 8 fritters on the prepared baking sheet, patting them out into disks about ½ inch thick. Generously spray the tops of the fritters with oil. Bake for 15 minutes, then flip the fritters and bake for another 5 to 10 minutes, until browned and cooked through.

Continued >

4. **Make the sauce.** Meanwhile, combine the yogurt, dill, garlic, salt, and black pepper in a food processor and purée until smooth. Taste and adjust the salt as needed. Scrape into a bowl.

5. **Assemble the bowls.** Divide the spinach among four shallow bowls. Top each bowl with 2 fritters and drizzle with sauce. Serve hot.

Per Serving: *Calories: 293; Fat: 21g; Protein: 15g; Total Carbs: 17g; Fiber: 5g; Sodium: 996mg; Iron: 3mg*

Spicy Curry Pancakes with Quick Slaw

Think of these pancakes like flatbread, perfect for scooping up bites of spicy-sweet slaw. Before you put a whole jalapeño in the batter, taste to see just how hot it is. Jalapeño heat really varies by season, so you might end up using a little or a lot, depending on how spicy you want the crepes to be.

SERVES 4

Active time: 20 minutes
Total time: 25 minutes

LOW-CARB, VEGETARIAN

FOR THE SLAW

½ cup Mayonnaise (page 166) or store-bought Paleo mayonnaise

1 tablespoon apple cider vinegar

1 tablespoon maple syrup

1 teaspoon sriracha

½ teaspoon salt

4 cups shredded cabbage

4 scallions, white and green parts, thinly sliced

2 tablespoons raisins (optional)

Freshly ground black pepper

FOR THE PANCAKES

½ cup almond flour

½ cup arrowroot starch

1 cup canned full-fat coconut milk

½ cup chopped fresh cilantro

¼ cup finely chopped shallot

1 jalapeño, seeded (if desired) and minced

2 teaspoons curry powder

1 teaspoon sea salt

Freshly ground black pepper

Avocado oil, for frying

1. **Make the slaw.** In a small bowl, stir together the mayonnaise, vinegar, maple syrup, sriracha, and salt in a small bowl. In a medium bowl, combine the cabbage, scallions, and raisins (if using). Pour the dressing over and toss to coat. Taste and add more salt as needed and finish with several grinds of pepper. Refrigerate while you fry the pancakes.

2. **Make the pancakes.** In a medium bowl, stir together the almond flour, arrowroot, coconut milk, cilantro, shallot, jalapeño, curry powder, salt, and a few grinds of pepper. Heat ¼ inch of oil in a 12-inch nonstick skillet over medium heat. When the oil is hot, pour about ¼ cup of the batter on one side of the pan, then another ¼ cup on the other side.

Continued >

Fry the 2 pancakes until crisp on the bottom, 2 to 3 minutes, then flip and fry until crisp on the other side, about 2 minutes more. Transfer to a large plate. Fry the remaining pancakes in the same manner, adding more oil as needed.

3. **Serve.** Divide the slaw among four dinner plates. Serve with the warm pancakes—you can use them like flatbread to eat the slaw.

SMART SHOPPING: If you buy Primal Kitchen's chipotle-lime mayonnaise, skip the sriracha.

COOKING HACK: Make quick work of shredding the cabbage by using a mandoline or food processor. Or pick up a bag of shredded coleslaw mix in the produce department.

Per Serving *(without raisins): Calories: 471; Fat: 45g; Protein: 4g; Total Carbs: 17g; Fiber: 3g; Sodium: 987mg; Iron: 7mg*

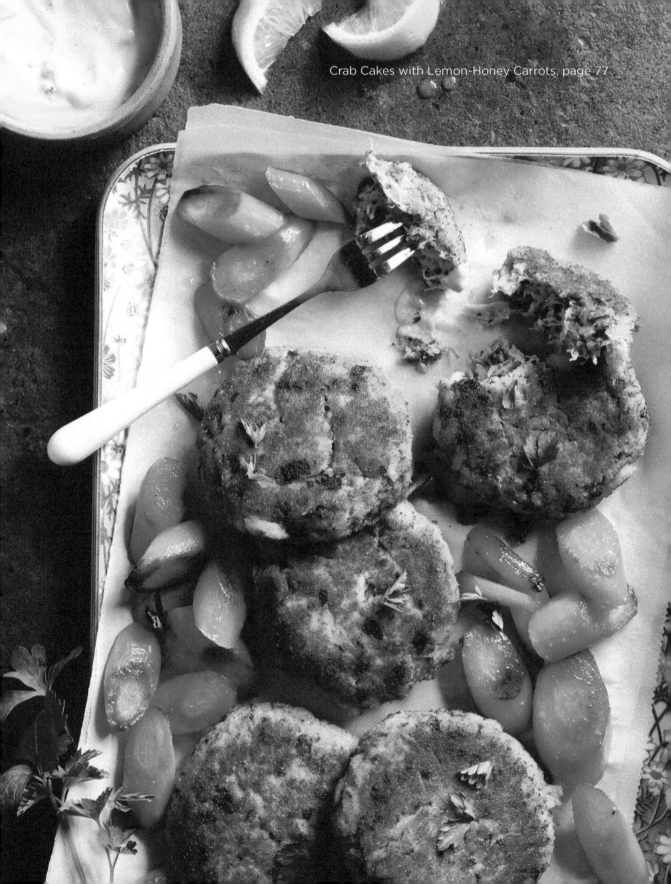

Crab Cakes with Lemon-Honey Carrots, page 77

Seafood

Clam, Halibut, and Kale Chowder

To me, no soup is cozier and more warming than a creamy chowder chock-full of bacon and potatoes. Given that winter lasts for a long time in Minnesota, I make chowder several times a year. I always keep a stash of canned clams and clam juice on hand so I can make this quickly.

SERVES 4 TO 6

Active time: 25 minutes
Total time: 30 minutes

1 cup raw cashews

1 cup hot water

4 (6.5-ounce) cans minced clams

2 (8-ounce) bottles clam juice

1 cup cool water

4 thick-cut bacon slices, finely chopped

1 medium yellow onion, finely chopped

2 cups thinly sliced lacinato kale leaves, center ribs removed

2 large red potatoes, peeled and cut into ¼-inch dice

¼ teaspoon dried thyme

1 (8-ounce) halibut fillet, cut into ½-inch pieces

2 tablespoons minced fresh parsley

Sea salt

Freshly ground black pepper

1. **Get ready.** Put the cashews and hot water in a blender. Set aside to soak. Open the cans of clams and drain them over a medium bowl, reserving the clams and their broth separately. Add the clam juice and the cool water to the clam broth. Set aside.

2. **Cook the bacon and vegetables.** In a large saucepan, fry the bacon over medium heat until the fat renders and the bacon is crisp, about 6 minutes. Add the onion and cook, stirring occasionally, until softened, about 5 minutes. Add the kale and sauté until wilted, about 5 minutes.

3. **Simmer the broth and potatoes.** Gradually stir in the reserved clam broth mixture. Add the potatoes and thyme, then simmer until the potatoes are tender, about 10 minutes.

4. **Purée the cashews.** While the broth simmers, blend the cashews and water, starting on low and increasing the speed until very smooth and creamy. Set aside.

5. **Finish and serve the chowder.** When the potatoes are tender, add the halibut to the broth and simmer until just cooked through, about 3 minutes. Add the reserved clams, cashew purée, and

parsley. Taste and season with salt as needed. Add a few grinds of pepper. Bring just to a simmer, then remove from the heat. Serve immediately.

SIMPLE SWAP: Instead of halibut, feel free to use cod, salmon, or your other favorite firm-fleshed fish.

Per Serving: *Calories: 527; Fat: 32g; Protein: 20g; Total Carbs: 44g; Fiber: 5g; Sodium: 796mg; Iron: 5mg*

Manhattan Crab Chowder

You know when you come home from a trip—starving—and have nothing to make for dinner? Stock up on the pantry staples that make up most of this easy chowder and that will never happen again. In 30 minutes, you'll be enjoying a hearty bowl of this classic tomato-based chowder.

SERVES 4

Active time: 25 minutes
Total time: 30 minutes

....
NUT-FREE

4 thick-cut bacon slices, cut into ½-inch pieces

1 medium yellow onion, finely chopped

½ celery stalk, finely chopped

2 garlic cloves, minced

1 teaspoon dried oregano

3 (8-ounce) bottles clam juice

1 tablespoon freshly squeezed lemon juice

2 large Yukon Gold potatoes, cut into ¼-inch dice

1 (14.5-ounce) can diced tomatoes

2 (6-ounce) cans crabmeat, drained

Sea salt

Freshly ground black pepper

½ cup chopped fresh parsley, for garnish

1. **Fry the bacon and vegetables.** In a large saucepan, fry the bacon over medium heat until the fat renders and the bacon is crisp, about 6 minutes. Add the onion and celery, reduce the heat to low, cover, and cook until softened, about 10 minutes. Add the garlic and oregano and sauté until fragrant, about 1 minute.

2. **Prepare the broth.** Add the clam juice, lemon juice, and potatoes. Bring to a boil over medium-high heat, reduce the heat to low, and simmer until the potatoes are almost tender, 8 to 10 minutes. Using a spoon, smash a few potatoes against the side of the pot to thicken the broth. Add the tomatoes with their juice, bring back to a simmer, and cook for 5 minutes.

3. **Finish the chowder and serve.** Remove the pan from the heat, stir in the crabmeat, and season with salt and pepper. Stir in the parsley and serve.

Per Serving: *Calories: 376; Fat: 12g; Protein: 27g; Total Carbs: 41g; Fiber: 7g; Sodium: 842mg; Iron: 3mg*

Crab Cakes with Lemon-Honey Carrots

Crab cakes might seem fussy, but they're actually very simple to make. You can make these with standard-issue canned crabmeat, but for super special crab cakes, buy pasteurized lump crabmeat, which is sold refrigerated in plastic containers and has a texture and flavor quite close to fresh crab, but with a longer shelf life. Coconut flour gives a lovely crust, and don't worry—it doesn't taste coconutty here.

SERVES 4

Active time: 25 minutes
Total time: 30 minutes

....
LOW-CARB

FOR THE SAUCE

2 tablespoons Mayonnaise (page 166) or store-bought Paleo mayonnaise

2 tablespoons Dijon mustard

FOR THE CRAB CAKES

1 (1-pound) container pasteurized lump crabmeat

⅓ cup almond flour

2 scallions, white and green parts, minced

¼ cup minced fresh parsley

2 teaspoons Old Bay seasoning

1 large egg, lightly beaten

3 tablespoons Mayonnaise (page 166) or store-bought Paleo mayonnaise

Freshly ground black pepper

FOR THE CARROTS

8 medium carrots, peeled and cut on a diagonal into ½-inch pieces

2 tablespoons avocado oil

¼ teaspoon sea salt

1 tablespoon honey

2 teaspoons freshly squeezed lemon juice

FOR FRYING

½ cup coconut flour

4 tablespoons avocado oil

1. **Get ready.** Preheat the oven to 425°F. Line two rimmed baking sheets with parchment paper or aluminum foil.

2. **Make the sauce.** In a small bowl, stir together the mayonnaise and mustard. Set aside.

3. **Prepare the crab cakes.** In a large bowl, combine the crab, almond flour, scallions, parsley, Old Bay, egg, mayonnaise, and several grinds of pepper. Mix gently. Form the mixture into 8 even patties, about 1 inch thick, and set them on one of the prepared baking sheets. When all the patties are formed, set the baking sheet in the refrigerator for a few minutes while you prepare the carrots.

Continued >

4. **Roast the carrots.** In a medium bowl, toss the carrots with the oil and salt. Spread them out on the other prepared baking sheet (reserve the bowl) and roast for 15 minutes. Turn the carrots and roast for another 5 to 10 minutes, until nicely browned. Meanwhile, in a small bowl, stir together the honey and lemon juice. When the carrots are done, return them to the reserved bowl, drizzle with the honey mixture, and toss to coat. Season with more salt as needed. Keep warm.

5. **Fry the crab cakes.** While the carrots are roasting, put the coconut flour on a large plate. Remove the crab cakes from the refrigerator. Lightly dredge them in the coconut flour, brushing away any clumps. Heat 2 tablespoons of oil in a 10-inch nonstick skillet over medium heat. When the oil is hot, fry a few crab cakes at a time until nicely browned, about 4 minutes per side. Use the remaining 2 tablespoons of oil as needed. Transfer to a paper towel–lined platter as you go.

6. **Serve.** Divide the carrots among four dinner plates. Add 2 crab cakes to each plate and serve with the sauce on the side.

Per Serving: *Calories: 535; Fat: 42g; Protein: 27g; Total Carbs: 14g; Fiber: 2g; Sodium: 777mg; Iron: 3mg*

Spicy Shrimp, Chorizo, and Spinach Soup

This spicy sausage soup requires just a little chopping and only one pot, but it delivers tons of spicy, filling flavor. If you can't find dried chorizo, you can substitute fresh—just brown it with the vegetables.

SERVES 4

Active time: 25 minutes
Total time: 30 minutes

....

LOW-CARB, NUT-FREE, ONE-PAN

2 tablespoons avocado oil

1 medium yellow onion, cut into ¼-inch dice

1 celery stalk, finely chopped

1 medium carrot, peeled and cut into ¼-inch dice

1 large red potato, peeled and cut into ½-inch dice

6 ounces dry-cured chorizo, cut into ½-inch dice

1 teaspoon smoked paprika

½ teaspoon sea salt

1 (14-ounce) can diced tomatoes, preferably fire-roasted

4 cups Rich Chicken Broth (page 158) or store-bought chicken broth

1 pound medium or large shrimp, peeled, deveined, and cut into ½-inch pieces

4 cups coarsely chopped spinach leaves, stems removed

1 tablespoon freshly squeezed lemon juice

Freshly ground black pepper

1. **Prepare the broth.** Heat the oil in a Dutch oven over medium heat. When the oil is hot, add the onion, celery, carrot, potato, chorizo, paprika, and salt. Sauté, stirring frequently, until the vegetables soften, about 10 minutes. Add the tomatoes with their juice and the broth and bring to a boil. Turn the heat to medium-low and simmer for 10 minutes.

2. **Finish the soup and serve.** Add the shrimp and spinach to the pan. Bring the broth back to a simmer, stirring a few times, and cook for 1 to 2 minutes, until the shrimp is pink and the spinach is wilted. Stir in the lemon juice. Season the soup with salt and a few grinds of pepper and serve.

SERVING SUGGESTION: Diced avocado makes a terrific garnish for this soup.

COOKING HACK: Did you know that adding acid (think lemon juice or vinegar) to a dish diminishes the taste of salt? Keep that trick up your sleeve if you oversalt a dish. And remember to season a dish with salt *after* adding acid.

Per Serving: Calories: 472; Fat: 27g; Protein: 30g; Total Carbs: 28g; Fiber: 5g; Sodium: 998mg; Iron: 3mg

Slow-Cooked Halibut with Swiss Chard and Yogurt Dressing

Cooking fish slowly yields an extra tender result in this warm salad. It's important to eat greens with some fat to properly absorb the fat-soluble nutrients, so don't skimp on the olive oil when sautéing the Swiss chard. Tangy, creamy coconut yogurt dressing ties it all together beautifully.

SERVES 4

Active time: 15 minutes
Total time: 20 minutes

5 INGREDIENTS, LOW-CARB, NUT-FREE, ONE-PAN

FOR THE DRESSING

⅓ cup plain coconut yogurt

2 tablespoons apple cider vinegar

1 tablespoon avocado oil

½ teaspoon sea salt

Freshly ground black pepper

FOR THE HALIBUT AND CHARD

4 (4-ounce) skinless halibut fillets

Sea salt

2 tablespoons extra-virgin olive oil, plus more as needed

8 cups thinly sliced Swiss chard leaves, center ribs removed

2 garlic cloves, very thinly sliced

1 cup lightly torn fresh tender herbs, such as basil, chervil, tarragon, and/or parsley

1. **Make the dressing.** Combine the yogurt, vinegar, oil, salt, and pepper in a jar, cover, and shake to combine. Taste and adjust the seasoning as needed. Set aside.

2. **Make the halibut.** Pat the halibut fillets dry with a paper towel and sprinkle both sides with a bit of salt. Heat the oil in a 12-inch nonstick skillet over the lowest heat possible. When the oil is hot, add the fish to the pan. Cook the fish very gently for 3 minutes—there should be no sizzling—then turn it over with a spatula. Continue cooking for another 3 minutes, then make a small cut in the thickest part of one of the fillets and check—if it's mostly cooked through with just a hint of translucence at the center, it's done. Transfer the fish to a plate.

3. **Make the chard.** Set the same skillet over medium heat. If the pan is dry, add a drizzle of oil. Add the chard and a pinch of salt. Sauté, stirring a few times, until the chard begins to wilt. Add the garlic and sauté for 2 to 3 minutes more, until the chard is tender. Transfer the chard to a bowl.

4. **Finish the dish.** Toss the chard with the herbs and divide among four shallow bowls. Gently break the halibut into large pieces and divide among the bowls, nestling the fish alongside the greens. Lightly drizzle the chard and halibut with the dressing. Finish with a sprinkle of salt and serve.

SERVING TIP: This is a naturally low-carbohydrate dish. Serve with boiled or roasted new potatoes to add a starch.

Per Serving: *Calories: 356; Fat: 30g; Protein: 18g; Total Carbs: 4g; Fiber: 1g; Sodium: 415mg; Iron: 3mg*

Panfried Trout with Steamed Broccoli

The nutty crust on this trout dish makes it restaurant worthy. It also makes it pretty rich, so simply steamed broccoli alongside is the perfect foil. Don't skip the lemon finish—it really pulls everything together and makes the broccoli pop. If you want to add a starch to the meal, a baked sweet potato would go especially well.

SERVES 4

Active time: 20 minutes
Total time: 20 minutes

....
LOW-CARB

1½ cups raw walnuts or pecans

1 garlic clove, chopped

1 teaspoon sea salt

1 large egg

4 tablespoons ghee or avocado
   oil, divided

4 (5-ounce) trout fillets

1 head broccoli, cut into florets

1 lemon, cut into 4 wedges, for garnish

1. **Get ready.** Pour 1 inch of water into a pot and add a steamer basket. Set over medium-low heat so that water heats while you cook the trout.

2. **Prepare the trout coating.** Combine the walnuts, garlic, and salt in a food processor. Pulse until the nuts are the size of small pebbles—you want some texture, but not large pieces. Transfer to a plate. Lightly beat the egg in a pie plate or shallow bowl.

3. **Coat and fry the trout.** Heat 2 tablespoons of ghee in a 10-inch nonstick skillet over medium heat. While the ghee heats, dip 2 of the trout fillets first in egg and then in the walnuts, pressing down so the walnuts stick to the fish. You only need to coat one side of the fish in nuts. When the ghee is hot, add 2 of the fillets, nut-side down, and fry, pressing down on the fish a few times so the coating adheres. Cook for 3 to 4 minutes per side, until nicely crisp. Transfer to two dinner plates. Repeat with the remaining 2 tablespoons of ghee and trout fillets.

4. **Steam the broccoli.** While the trout cooks, turn the heat to high under the pot of water. When the water boils, fill the steamer basket with the broccoli. Cover and steam for 5 to 6 minutes, to your desired doneness.

5. **Finish the dish and serve.** Divide the broccoli among the plates. Top the trout and broccoli with squeezes of lemon and a sprinkle of salt and serve.

SERVING SUGGESTION: If you have Chimichurri (see page 160) on hand, a spoonful would be amazing over the broccoli and/or trout.

SIMPLE SWAP: To make this dish nut-free, either substitute pepitas for the nuts or skip the nut coating entirely and just cook the seasoned trout in ghee or avocado oil.

COOKING HACK: Did you know you can steam broccoli in the microwave? Pour enough water into a large microwave-safe bowl to just cover the bottom. Add broccoli and cover with plastic wrap. Cook on high for 3 to 5 minutes, to your desired doneness.

Per Serving: *Calories: 632; Fat: 48g; Protein: 41g; Total Carbs: 13g; Fiber: 5g; Sodium: 716mg; Iron: 5mg*

Fish Tacos with Roasted Pineapple

Pineapple roasted with chiles, oil, and salt turns into a spicy, caramelized dream. It's so flavorful, you don't have to fuss too much with the fish to make memorable tacos. Instead of grilling or frying, I prefer to bake the fish in foil packets to keep it moist. My favorite Paleo tortillas are Siete Foods' cassava and coconut tortillas.

SERVES 4

Active time: 20 minutes
Total time: 25 minutes

....
NUT-FREE

FOR THE PINEAPPLE

2 cups ½-inch pineapple chunks

1 jalapeño, seeded (if desired) and minced

1 tablespoon avocado oil

¼ teaspoon sea salt

¼ cup chopped fresh cilantro

FOR THE FISH

4 (4-ounce) firm-fleshed white fish fillets, such as tilapia, cod, or halibut

Sea salt

2 tablespoons freshly squeezed lime juice

2 tablespoons avocado oil

1 garlic clove, minced

1 teaspoon dried oregano

FOR THE TACOS

8 Plantain Tortillas (page 159) or store-bought Paleo tortillas

1 cup thinly sliced red cabbage, for garnish

1 avocado, pitted, peeled, and sliced, for garnish

¼ cup chopped sweet onion (or red onion, if you prefer more bite), for garnish

Hot sauce, for serving

1. **Get ready.** Preheat the oven to 400°F. Arrange two racks toward the center of the oven. Line a rimmed baking sheet with parchment paper or aluminum foil.

2. **Prepare the pineapple.** In a medium bowl, toss together the pineapple, jalapeño, oil, and salt. Spread out the pineapple on the prepared baking sheet. Bake for 10 minutes, setting a timer.

3. **Prepare the fish.** Meanwhile, tear off 4 (12-inch) pieces of aluminum foil. Place 2 fillets side-by-side on one piece and 2 fillets on another piece. Season the fish with salt. In a small bowl, stir together the lime juice, oil, garlic, and oregano. Spoon the mixture over the fish fillets. Place another piece of foil on top of each and fold up all the edges to create two sealed packets. Place the packets on another baking sheet.

4. **Bake the fish.** When the timer goes off, stir the pineapple then return it to the oven. At the same time, put the baking sheet with the fish packets in the oven. Wrap the tortillas in foil and add them to the oven as well. Bake until the pineapple is brown and caramelized and the fish is cooked through, 10 minutes for thinner fillets or 15 minutes for thicker fillets.

5. **Finish the dish.** Transfer the pineapple to a bowl and stir in the cilantro. Break the fish into bite-size pieces and sprinkle with a bit more salt as needed. Set out the warm tortillas, cabbage, avocado, onion, and hot sauce and serve.

SMART SHOPPING: You can buy peeled and cored fresh pineapple or pineapple chunks in the produce section of most grocery stores.

Per Serving: *Calories: 513; Fat: 20g; Protein: 24g; Total Carbs: 64g; Fiber: 11g; Sodium: 693mg; Iron: 2mg*

Cold Noodle Salad with Glazed Salmon

The ingredient list looks a bit long, but this dish comes together in a snap. The chopping is simple and the rest is just stirring things together. If you have a garden bursting with basil and/or cilantro, you should tear the leaves and add to the salad—they'd be perfect!

SERVES 4

Active time: 20 minutes
Total time: 20 minutes

....
LOW-CARB, NUT-FREE

FOR THE SALAD

6 ounces sweet potato starch noodles (aka japchae or "glass" noodles)

2 cups thinly sliced lettuce

½ cup thinly sliced radishes

½ cup sliced scallions, white and green parts

½ cup torn fresh mint leaves

1 jalapeño, seeded (if desired) and minced

FOR THE DRESSING

¼ cup water

2 tablespoons fish sauce

1 tablespoon freshly squeezed lime juice

1 tablespoon maple syrup

2 garlic cloves, minced

1 teaspoon minced fresh ginger

FOR THE SALMON

4 (4-ounce) salmon fillets

Sea salt

1 tablespoon avocado oil

3 tablespoons coconut sugar

1. **Get ready.** Arrange an oven rack 8 inches from the broiler element. Preheat the broiler. Line a rimmed baking sheet with aluminum foil.

2. **Boil the noodles for the salad.** Fill a large pot with cold, salted water and bring to a boil over high heat. Add the noodles and cook according to the package directions; drain and rinse with cool water. If the noodles are very long, use scissors to trim them to 8 inches. Put the noodles in a large bowl.

3. **Make the dressing.** In a small bowl, whisk together the water, fish sauce, lime juice, maple syrup, garlic, and ginger.

4. **Prepare the salad.** Add half the dressing to the noodles and toss to coat. Add the lettuce, radishes, scallions, mint, and jalapeño and toss. Refrigerate while you prepare the salmon.

5. **Make the salmon.** Place the salmon fillets on the prepared baking sheet. Season lightly with salt. In a small bowl, stir together the oil and sugar. Spoon the glaze over the salmon and spread evenly. Broil the salmon to your desired doneness—about 5 minutes for thin fillets and 7 minutes for thicker fillets—watching closely as it broils.

6. **Finish the dish.** Divide the noodle salad among four shallow bowls. Top each with a salmon fillet. Drizzle more dressing over the top and serve immediately.

SIMPLE SWAPS: Choose halibut or cod in place of salmon.

Per Serving: *Calories: 287; Fat: 10g; Protein: 26g; Total Carbs: 22g; Fiber: 1g; Sodium: 845mg; Iron: 1mg*

Salmon Burgers in Lettuce with Smoky Roasted Potatoes

This is a fun twist on a traditional burger and fries. Canned salmon makes for very tasty burgers—the technique is exactly the same as the Crab Cakes (see page 77)—and what's better next to a burger than smoky, crispy potatoes? I love burgers in lettuce leaves, but if you're missing a bun sort of experience, Plantain Tortillas (see page 159) work nicely.

SERVES 4

Active time: 25 minutes
Total time: 30 minutes

FOR THE ROASTED POTATOES

2 pounds small red
   potatoes, quartered

3 tablespoons avocado oil

1 teaspoon smoked paprika

1 teaspoon sea salt

FOR THE SALMON BURGERS

3 (6-ounce) cans wild salmon, drained

⅓ cup almond flour

2 scallions, white and green
   parts, minced

1 large egg, lightly beaten

3 tablespoons Mayonnaise (page 166)
   or store-bought Paleo mayonnaise

½ teaspoon sea salt

Freshly ground black pepper

½ cup coconut flour

4 tablespoons avocado oil, divided

8 butter or iceberg lettuce leaves

1. **Get ready.** Preheat the oven to 450°F. Line two rimmed baking sheets with parchment paper or aluminum foil.

2. **Make the potatoes.** In a large bowl, toss the potatoes with the oil, paprika, and salt. Spread them out on one of the prepared baking sheets (wipe out and reserve the bowl). Roast for 15 minutes, stir, then roast for another 10 to 15 minutes, until the potatoes are crisp. Taste and add more salt as needed.

3. **Make the salmon burgers.** While the potatoes are roasting, in the reserved large bowl, combine the salmon, almond flour, scallions, egg, mayonnaise, salt, and several grinds of pepper. Mix gently. Form the mixture into 4 even patties, about 1 inch thick. Set them on the other prepared baking sheet. Put the coconut flour on a plate. Lightly dredge the salmon

burgers in the coconut flour, brushing away any clumps. Heat 2 tablespoons of oil in a 10-inch nonstick skillet over medium heat. When the oil is hot, fry a few salmon burgers at a time until nicely browned, about 4 minutes per side. Use the remaining 2 tablespoons of oil as needed. Transfer to a paper towel–lined platter as you go.

4. **Serve.** Divide the potatoes among four dinner plates. Serve the salmon burgers in the lettuce leaves alongside the potatoes.

SERVING SUGGESTION: Primal Kitchen makes a delicious Paleo ketchup, which would be great with both the potatoes and the burgers. Alternatively—or also!—you could use additional mayonnaise on the burger and/or for dipping the potatoes. A slice of sweet onion with the burger is really nice.

Per Serving: *Calories: 649; Fat: 38g; Protein: 31g; Total Carbs: 45g; Fiber: 5g; Sodium: 992mg; Iron: 4mg*

Classic Tuna Diner Salad

I call this a classic diner salad because it is in spirit—although the diner salads I ate growing up didn't have avocado, fresh herbs, or jammy eggs! I loved those salads anyhow, so I really adore this version, with better ingredients and plenty of zing. If you want a no-cook meal, simply skip the eggs.

SERVES 4

Active time: 20 minutes
Total time: 20 minutes

....

LOW-CARB, NUT-FREE

FOR THE SALAD

4 large eggs

4 cups salad greens

4 radishes, thinly sliced

4 scallions, white and green parts, thinly sliced

3 tablespoons chopped fresh dill

1 large avocado, pitted and peeled, half sliced and half mashed

FOR THE TUNA

3 (5-ounce) cans albacore tuna, drained

⅓ cup Mayonnaise (page 166) or store-bought Paleo mayonnaise

⅓ cup finely chopped sweet onion

⅓ cup finely chopped dill pickle

1 teaspoon freshly squeezed lemon juice

Sea salt

Freshly ground black pepper

FOR THE DRESSING AND SERVING

2 tablespoons extra-virgin olive oil

1 tablespoon freshly squeezed lemon juice

Sea salt

Freshly ground black pepper

1. **Boil the eggs for the salad.** Fill a small saucepan with water and bring to a boil over high heat. Gently add the eggs, turn the heat to medium, and cook for 7 to 8 minutes (7 minutes for firm yolks with runny centers, 8 minutes for jammy eggs). Use tongs or a slotted spoon to transfer the eggs to a bowl of cold water.

2. **Prepare the salad.** Divide the salad greens, radishes, scallions, and dill among four shallow bowls. Top with the avocado slices (reserve the mashed avocado for the tuna). Set aside.

3. **Prepare the tuna.** In a medium bowl, combine the tuna, mashed avocado, mayonnaise, onion, pickle, and lemon juice. Stir to combine. Season with salt and pepper.

4. **Make the dressing and serve.** In a small bowl, whisk together the olive oil, lemon juice, and a pinch of salt. Drizzle over the salad greens. Divide the tuna salad among the salads. (Use an ice cream scoop if you really want to be retro!) Peel and halve the eggs and divide among the bowls. Sprinkle the eggs with a bit of salt. Grind pepper over the salads and serve.

Per Serving: *Calories: 451; Fat: 33g; Protein: 29g; Total Carbs: 11g; Fiber: 6g; Sodium: 646mg; Iron: 5mg*

Pasta with White Clam Sauce

Spaghetti with clam sauce was a college staple for me. I lived alone for the first time in my life, so I could experiment with cooking to my heart's content—or to my limited budget's content! Splurging on canned clams was a delightful upgrade to my usual pasta dishes.

SERVES 2 TO 4

Active time: 20 minutes
Total time: 20 minutes

. . . .
LOW-CARB, NUT-FREE

8 ounces sweet potato starch noodles (aka japchae or "glass" noodles)

2 (6-ounce) cans minced clams

¼ cup extra-virgin olive oil

4 garlic cloves, minced

⅛ teaspoon red pepper flakes

½ cup dry white wine

1 teaspoon freshly squeezed lemon juice

¼ cup chopped fresh parsley

Freshly ground black pepper

1. **Boil the noodles.** Bring a large pot of salted water to a boil over high heat. Add the noodles and cook according to the package directions; drain and rinse with cool water. If the noodles are very long, use scissors to trim them to 8 inches.

2. **Prepare the sauce.** Open the cans of clams and drain them over a medium bowl, reserving the clams and their broth separately. Heat the oil in a 12-inch nonstick skillet over medium heat. When the oil is hot, add the garlic and red pepper flakes and sauté for 3 minutes. Add the reserved clam broth and white wine and bring to a boil. Boil the sauce until reduced to about ½ cup, 3 to 4 minutes. Turn the heat to low.

3. **Finish the noodles and serve.** Add the reserved clams, lemon juice, and parsley to the pan, then add the noodles. Grind black pepper over the noodles and toss until combined and heated through. Serve immediately.

SERVING SUGGESTION: To fill out the meal, serve with a simple green salad dressed with lemony vinaigrette.

SIMPLE SWAP: If you prefer a more traditional pasta feel, Cappello's Paleo spaghetti is terrific in this recipe.

Per Serving: Calories: 252; Fat: 14g; Protein: 2g; Total Carbs: 25g; Fiber: 1g; Sodium: 326mg; Iron: <1mg

Blackened Snapper with Mustard Greens

Blackened fish paired with brothy greens is a classic combination, and for good reason—they taste fantastic together. "Blackened" is the effect of frying spice-coated fish until the spices are deeply browned. If you want extra spiciness, add a pinch of cayenne to the spice rub. Make sure to serve in a shallow bowl so you don't lose any of the delectable pan juices.

SERVES 4

Active time: 20 minutes
Total time: 20 minutes

....

LOW-CARB, NUT-FREE

FOR THE MUSTARD GREENS

2 tablespoons avocado oil

2 garlic cloves, thinly sliced

2 bunches mustard greens, ribs removed and leaves chopped (about 8 cups)

Sea salt

¼ cup Rich Chicken Broth (page 158) or store-bought chicken broth

1 tablespoon Dijon mustard

Freshly ground black pepper

FOR THE SNAPPER

1 teaspoon paprika

1 teaspoon dried thyme

1 teaspoon sea salt

½ teaspoon garlic powder

½ teaspoon freshly ground black pepper

4 (4-ounce) skin-on red snapper fillets

2 tablespoons avocado oil

1 lemon, cut into 8 wedges, for serving

1. **Cook the mustard greens.** Heat the oil in a Dutch oven or large high-sided skillet over medium heat. When the oil is hot, add the garlic and sauté for 3 minutes. Add the greens and a generous pinch of salt and stir to coat the greens with oil. Sauté the greens for 4 minutes, or until wilted. Add the broth and simmer for 5 minutes, or until the greens are tender. Stir in the mustard, season with additional salt and a few grinds of pepper, and keep warm while you cook the fish.

2. **Cook the snapper.** In a small bowl, combine the paprika, thyme, salt, garlic powder, and black pepper. Rub a generous amount of the seasoning mixture all over the fish (store any leftover spice in a jar for another use). Heat the oil in a 12-inch nonstick skillet over medium-high heat. When the oil is hot, lay the fish fillets, flesh-side down, and fry, without turning, until the bottom has a lovely dark brown ("blackened") crust,

Continued >

about 7 minutes. Flip the fish and press down with the back of a spatula to flatten. Fry for 3 to 4 minutes, until the fish is just cooked through.

3. **Serve.** Divide the greens among four shallow bowls, spooning the pan juices over them. Place a fillet alongside the greens. Squeeze lemon over the fish and serve.

Per Serving: *Calories: 254; Fat: 16g; Protein: 25g; Total Carbs: 3g; Fiber: 1g; Sodium: 461mg; Iron: <1mg*

Coconut Cod Stew with Roasted Squash

This creamy squash stew features tender coconut-perfumed fish. It's a complete meal as-is, but you could also serve cauliflower rice alongside.

SERVES 4

Active time: 25 minutes
Total time: 30 minutes

LOW-CARB, NUT-FREE

2 cups ½-inch diced, peeled, and seeded butternut squash

1 tablespoon coconut oil, melted

Sea salt

2 (13.5-ounce) cans full-fat coconut milk

1 medium yellow onion, finely chopped

2 garlic cloves, minced

2 tablespoons grated fresh ginger

1 tablespoon curry powder

½ cup water

2 tablespoons fish sauce

2 tablespoons coconut aminos

2 tablespoons maple syrup

1 pound cod, cut into 1-inch pieces

2 tablespoons lime juice

¼ cup chopped fresh cilantro

1. **Get ready.** Preheat the oven to 425°F. Line a rimmed baking sheet with parchment paper or aluminum foil.

2. **Roast the squash.** In a medium bowl, toss the squash with the coconut oil and a generous pinch of salt. Spread evenly on the prepared baking sheet and roast for 15 minutes. Stir the squash pieces and roast until tender and browned in spots, another 5 to 10 minutes. Set aside.

3. **Prepare the broth.** Spoon the fat from the top of the cans of coconut milk into a large saucepan. Set the pan over medium heat. When the fat is melted and hot, add the onion and sauté until softened and translucent, about 10 minutes. Add the garlic, ginger, and curry powder and sauté for 3 minutes. Mix in the remaining coconut milk, water, fish sauce, coconut aminos, and maple syrup and bring to a simmer. Turn the heat to low, cover, and simmer for 10 minutes.

4. **Cook the fish and serve.** Add the cod to the broth and simmer, uncovered, for 5 minutes, or until the cod is just cooked through. Stir in the lime juice. Adjust the seasoning with additional fish sauce, coconut aminos, and lime juice as needed. Stir in the roasted squash. Garnish with the cilantro and serve.

Per Serving: *Calories: 252; Fat: 14g; Protein: 2g; Total Carbs: 25g; Fiber: 1g; Sodium: 326mg; Iron: <1mg*

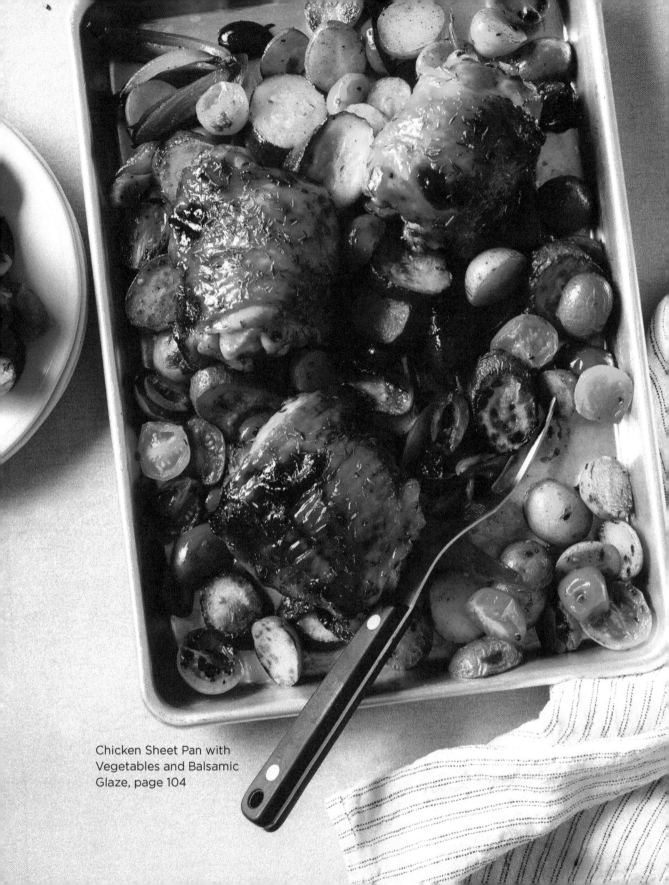

Chicken Sheet Pan with Vegetables and Balsamic Glaze, page 104

CHAPTER SIX

Poultry

Coconut Chicken Lettuce Wraps with Asparagus

I first created this recipe for my friend Joy's baby shower. Dairy was not agreeing with her, so I used coconut to add tenderness and flavor to ground chicken. Lettuce wraps are kid-friendly and so is this chicken filling—it's not spicy and it's very tender. If you love cilantro, feel free to add it, too—combined with the basil and mint, it provides yet another layers of freshness.

SERVES 4

Active time: 20 minutes
Total time: 20 minutes

....

LOW-CARB, NUT-FREE

1 pound asparagus, trimmed

1 tablespoon avocado oil

Sea salt

1 tablespoon coconut oil

1 small red onion, chopped

2 garlic cloves, minced

1 pound ground chicken

⅓ cup coconut milk

1 tablespoon fish sauce

2 tablespoons chopped fresh basil

2 tablespoons chopped fresh mint

1 tablespoon freshly squeezed
  lime juice

8 to 12 butter or iceberg lettuce leaves

1. **Get ready.** Preheat the oven to 425°F. Line a rimmed baking sheet with parchment paper or aluminum foil.

2. **Make the asparagus.** Put the asparagus on the prepared baking sheet. Drizzle with the avocado oil and sprinkle generously with salt. Toss to coat and arrange the asparagus in a single layer on the pan. Roast for 10 minutes, toss the asparagus, and roast for another 10 minutes, or until the asparagus is browned in spots.

3. **Make the chicken.** Meanwhile, heat the coconut oil in a 12-inch skillet over medium-high heat. When the oil is hot, add the onion and garlic and sauté for 5 minutes, or until the onion softens, then add the chicken. Using a spatula, break up the chicken as you sauté until the liquid is evaporated, about 9 minutes. Stir in the coconut milk and fish sauce. Cook, stirring occasionally, until the coconut milk is thickened, about 5 minutes. Stir in the basil, mint, and lime juice. Taste and adjust the seasoning as needed.

4. **Serve.** Divide the asparagus among four dinner plates. Spoon the chicken onto the lettuce leaves and eat with your hands. (I eat the asparagus with my hands, too, like fries, but that's totally up to you!)

SIMPLE SWAP: You can substitute ground pork for the ground chicken.

SERVING SUGGESTION: If you like, cauliflower rice works nicely in the wraps with the chicken.

Per Serving: *Calories: 294; Fat: 20g; Protein: 23g; Total Carbs: 8g; Fiber: 3g; Sodium: 325mg; Iron: 4mg*

Honey-Garlic Sticky Wings with Sesame Slaw

Put your blender to good use with this recipe—both the sauce for the wings and the slaw dressing get a quick purée. These heavenly chicken wings are roasted in the oven until crisp, then tossed with a sticky glaze and returned to the oven for just a few minutes until heated through.

SERVES 4

Active time: 25 minutes
Total time: 30 minutes

....
NUT-FREE

FOR THE WINGS

12 chicken wings, halved at the joint
(or 24 drummies/drummettes)

2 tablespoons avocado oil

1 teaspoon sea salt

FOR THE SAUCE

½ cup honey

¼ cup coconut aminos

¼ cup water

1 tablespoon Dijon mustard

2 teaspoons sriracha

4 garlic cloves, coarsely chopped

1 (3-inch) piece fresh ginger, peeled
and coarsely chopped

¼ teaspoon five-spice powder

FOR THE SLAW

2 tablespoons honey

2 tablespoons avocado oil

1 tablespoon toasted sesame oil

1 tablespoon apple cider vinegar

1 tablespoon coconut aminos

1 garlic clove, chopped

½ cup fresh cilantro leaves

8 ounces cabbage, shredded

1 tablespoon sesame seeds

Sea salt

1. **Get ready.** Arrange two racks toward the center of the oven. Preheat the oven to 450°F. Line two rimmed baking sheets with parchment paper or aluminum foil.

2. **Roast the wings.** In a large bowl, toss the chicken with the oil and salt until evenly coated. Arrange in a single layer on the prepared baking sheets. Roast for 10 minutes. Turn the wings over and roast for another 10 minutes.

3. **Make the sauce.** Meanwhile, combine the honey, coconut aminos, water, mustard, sriracha, garlic, ginger, and five-spice powder in a blender and blend until smooth. Pour the sauce into a Dutch oven and bring to a boil over medium-high heat (rinse the blender). Lower the heat

to medium-low and simmer until thickened and syrupy, about 4 to 5 minutes. Set aside.

4. **Make the slaw.** Combine the honey, avocado oil, sesame oil, vinegar, coconut aminos, garlic, and cilantro in the blender and purée until smooth. In a medium bowl, toss the cabbage with the honey-oil mixture. Add the sesame seeds and toss again. Season the slaw with salt as needed. Set aside.

5. **Finish the dish.** When the wings are done, add them to the sauce in the Dutch oven (reserve the baking sheets and keep the oven on) and toss to coat them. Spread the wings out on the baking sheets once more and bake for 5 minutes, or until sticky. Serve the wings with the slaw.

SMART SHOPPING: Buy packaged coleslaw mix to save time chopping cabbage.

SERVING SUGGESTION: If you have Ginger-Scallion Sauce (see page 161) on hand, it's great with these wings.

Per Serving: *Calories: 472; Fat: 21g; Protein: 23g; Total Carbs: 50g; Fiber: 2g; Sodium: 989mg; Iron: 2mg*

Chicken Piccata with Sautéed Swiss Chard

The signature tart lemon sauce of chicken piccata is so good with greens, I don't know why they're not always served together. This recipe calls for ghee, but you can substitute olive oil if you prefer. If you have extra time, mashed potatoes or cauliflower would be very welcome here.

SERVES 4

Active time: 20 minutes
Total time: 30 minutes

LOW-CARB, NUT-FREE, ONE-PAN

5 tablespoons extra-virgin olive oil, divided

1 pound Swiss chard, center ribs removed and leaves coarsely chopped

Sea salt

Freshly ground black pepper

4 boneless, skinless chicken breast halves (about 1 pound)

½ cup cassava flour

4 garlic cloves, coarsely chopped

½ cup Rich Chicken Broth (page 158) or store-bought chicken broth

2 tablespoons ghee or extra-virgin olive oil

2 tablespoons freshly squeezed lemon juice

2 tablespoons drained capers

1. **Prepare the chard.** Heat 1 tablespoon of oil in a 12-inch nonstick skillet over medium-high heat. When the oil is hot, add the chard, cover the pan, and let steam for 2 minutes. Uncover the pan and toss the chard. Continue tossing and stirring as it shrinks down, until the chard is wilted and tender and the liquid has evaporated, about 7 minutes total. Season the chard with salt and pepper. Scrape the chard into a bowl and keep warm (reserve the pan).

2. **Prepare the chicken.** Place each chicken between sheets of plastic wrap and use a meat mallet or rolling pin to pound into cutlets about ½ inch thick. Combine the cassava flour and 1 teaspoon of salt in a large plastic bag. Add the cutlets to the bag and shake around to coat with the flour.

3. **Fry the chicken.** Heat 2 tablespoons of oil in the reserved skillet over medium-high heat. When the oil is hot, remove 2 cutlets from the bag, shaking off the excess flour. Add the cutlets to the pan and fry until nicely browned and crisp on the bottom, about 3 minutes. Flip the chicken and cook until just cooked through, about 1 minute. Transfer to a plate. Repeat the process with the remaining

2 tablespoons of oil and remaining 2 chicken cutlets.

4. **Finish and serve.** Return the pan to the heat and add the garlic. Cook, stirring, until the garlic is starting to brown (being careful not to burn it). Add the broth, ghee, lemon juice, and capers and whisk continuously as the sauce simmers for 1 minute. Taste and add salt as needed. Add the chicken to the pan and simmer for 2 more minutes, or until the sauce is thickened a bit. Divide the chard among four shallow bowls. Top each with a chicken cutlet and spoon some sauce over the chicken and chard.

Per Serving: *Calories: 399; Fat: 26g; Protein: 30g; Total Carbs: 12g; Fiber: 3g; Sodium: 894mg; Iron: 4mg*

Chicken Sheet Pan with Vegetables and Balsamic Glaze

Sheet pan dinners are a flavorful way to get dinner on the table fast. The basic formula is protein + vegetables + seasoning + a delicious glaze or sauce. I've given you a basic idea here, but I promise that after you get the hang of this recipe, you'll start improvising with whatever flavors that you're craving.

SERVES 4

Active time: 15 minutes
Total time: 30 minutes

....
NUT-FREE

FOR THE GLAZE

¼ cup balsamic vinegar

3 tablespoons extra-virgin olive oil

2 tablespoons maple syrup

1 tablespoon Dijon mustard

2 garlic cloves, minced

1 teaspoon dried thyme

FOR THE CHICKEN AND VEGETABLES

1 pound bone-in, skin-on chicken thighs

1 pound small new potatoes, quartered

1 pound zucchini, cut into ½-inch slices

½ medium red onion, cut into ½-inch slices

1 cup cherry tomatoes, halved

12 kalamata olives, pitted and halved

1 teaspoon sea salt

Freshly ground black pepper

1. **Get ready.** Preheat the oven to 425°F. Line a rimmed baking sheet with parchment paper or aluminum foil.

2. **Make the glaze.** In a large bowl, whisk together the vinegar, olive oil, maple syrup, mustard, garlic, and thyme.

3. **Make the chicken and vegetables.** Add the chicken, potatoes, zucchini, onion, tomatoes, olives, and salt to the bowl with the glaze and stir to coat. Pour the chicken and vegetables out onto the prepared baking sheet and spread the vegetables out in a single layer. Place the chicken thighs, skin-side up, on top of the vegetables. Season the chicken thighs with salt.

4. **Finish the dish.** Roast for 15 minutes. Turn the vegetables (leave the chicken thighs skin-side up) and roast for 5 to 10 more minutes, until everything is nicely browned. Grind some pepper on top and serve.

SIMPLE SWAP: Sub 1-inch broccoli or cauliflower florets or halved Brussels sprouts for the zucchini.

Per Serving: *Calories: 691; Fat: 44g; Protein: 38g; Total Carbs: 36g; Fiber: 5g; Sodium: 924mg; Iron: 4mg*

Turkey Burgers with Rutabaga Fries

Ketchup, coconut aminos, and smoked paprika mixed into ground turkey give a hint of barbecue flavor to these juicy burgers. If you haven't worked with rutabaga before, the peel is tough and needs to be pared away, but the flesh makes terrific, low-carb fries. Primal Kitchen makes a no-sugar Paleo ketchup that I actually like better than traditional ketchup.

SERVES 4

Active time: 25 minutes
Total time: 25 minutes

....

LOW-CARB, NUT-FREE

FOR THE FRIES

2 (12-ounce) rutabagas, peeled and cut into ½-inch "fries"

3 tablespoons avocado oil

½ teaspoon garlic powder

½ teaspoon sea salt

Freshly ground black pepper

FOR THE BURGERS

1 pound ground turkey

2 scallions, white and green parts, minced

2 tablespoons Paleo ketchup

1 tablespoon coconut aminos

2 teaspoons arrowroot starch

½ teaspoon smoked paprika

1 teaspoon sea salt

Freshly ground black pepper

1 tablespoon avocado oil

16 butter or iceberg lettuce leaves

FOR THE OPTIONAL GARNISHES

Cashew Cheese (page 163)

Tomato slices

Pickled Red Onions (page 165)

Pickle slices

Mayonnaise (page 166) or store-bought Paleo mayonnaise

Mustard

Paleo ketchup

1. **Get ready.** Preheat the oven to 425°F. Line a rimmed baking sheet with parchment paper or aluminum foil and place a wire rack on the baking sheet.

2. **Prepare the fries.** In a large bowl, toss the rutabaga fries with the oil, garlic powder, salt, and several grinds of pepper. Arrange the fries on the rack on the baking sheet (reserve the bowl). Roast for 20 to 25 minutes, until the fries are browned.

3. **Prepare the burgers.** Meanwhile, in the reserved bowl, combine the turkey, scallions, ketchup, coconut

Continued >

aminos, arrowroot, smoked paprika, salt, and several grinds of pepper. Using your hands, mix until all the seasonings are incorporated into the meat. Gently form the mixture into 4 even patties, pressing a slight indentation into the center of each burger to help them cook more evenly.

4. **Fry the burgers.** Heat the oil in a 12-inch nonstick skillet over medium-high heat. When the oil is hot, add the patties and fry for 5 minutes. Flip the patties and fry for another 5 minutes, or until cooked through.

5. **Finish the dish.** Stack 2 lettuce leaves on each dinner plate. Top each with a burger, then with 2 more lettuce leaves. Divide the fries among the plates and serve with your choice of garnishes.

Per Serving *(without garnish): Calories: 315; Fat: 20g; Protein: 24g; Total Carbs: 13g; Fiber: 3g; Sodium: 936mg; Iron: 2mg*

Loaded Turkey Nachos

I'll admit that these are unconventional nachos. First off, there's (of course) no cheese, but I don't think you'll miss it. There's so much else going on, namely flavorful taco meat and all the other great toppings. Second, I suggest a dab of ketchup in the turkey—sounds odd, but it adds moisture and depth to the meat. And third, you don't have to bake the nachos after assembling them (again, no cheese), which saves time! I like Siete's grain-free tortilla chips, which are widely available in natural grocery stores and online.

SERVES 4

Active time: 20 minutes
Total time: 20 minutes
......
NUT-FREE, ONE-PAN

FOR THE TACO MEAT

1 tablespoon avocado oil

1 small yellow onion, finely chopped

1 pound ground turkey

1 teaspoon cumin

1 teaspoon chili powder

1 teaspoon dried oregano

1 teaspoon garlic powder

1 teaspoon sea salt

2 tablespoons Paleo ketchup

2 tablespoons water

1 teaspoon arrowroot starch

FOR THE NACHOS

1 (5-ounce) bag grain-free tortillas chips

2 cups shredded iceberg lettuce

2 tablespoons sliced black olives

1 jalapeño, seeded (if desired) and thinly sliced

Pickled Red Onions (page 165)

1 avocado, pitted, peeled, and diced

Hot sauce, for drizzling

1. **Cook the taco meat.** Heat the oil in a 12-inch skillet over medium-high heat. When the oil is hot, add the onion and cook until starting to brown, about 7 minutes. Turn the heat to medium and add the turkey, cumin, chili powder, oregano, garlic powder, and salt. Using a spatula, break up the turkey, stirring in the spices as it browns. When the turkey is no longer pink, stir in the ketchup and water and continue stirring until the liquid is evaporated. Stir in the arrowroot and cook for 1 minute. Remove the pan from the heat.

2. **Assemble the nachos and serve.** Spread the chips on a large platter. Top evenly with the taco meat. Scatter the lettuce, olives, jalapeño, pickled onions, and avocado over the nachos. Drizzle with hot sauce and serve immediately.

Continued >

SERVING SUGGESTIONS: If you have time, make the cashew crema from the Spicy Roasted Cauliflower Tacos (see page 60) of this book and drizzle over the nachos. You can also add chopped, ripe tomato and/or pepitas, if you like.

COOKING HACK: Substitute packaged taco mix for the cumin, chili powder, oregano, garlic powder, and salt. Primal Palate makes an excellent Paleo taco seasoning.

Per Serving: *Calories: 491; Fat: 28g; Protein: 27g; Total Carbs: 36g; Fiber: 7g; Sodium: 894mg; Iron: 3mg*

Weeknight Chicken Chili

Using ground chicken makes this creamy chili come together quickly. It contains sweet potato for starch as well as a hint of sweetness, but you can use Yukon Gold potatoes if you like.

SERVES 4

Active time: 15 minutes
Total time: 25 minutes

....

LOW-CARB, NUT-FREE, ONE-PAN

FOR THE CHILI

1 tablespoon extra-virgin olive oil

1 medium white onion, finely chopped

1 pound ground chicken

2 garlic cloves, minced

1 jalapeño, seeded (if desired) and finely chopped

1 tablespoon cassava flour

1 tablespoon ground cumin

Sea salt

1 medium sweet potato, peeled and cut into ½-inch dice (about 1 cup)

4 cups Rich Chicken Broth (page 158) or store-bought chicken broth

½ cup canned full-fat coconut milk

3 (4.5-ounce) cans chopped green chiles

FOR THE OPTIONAL GARNISHES

1 avocado, pitted, peeled, and diced

¼ cup chopped fresh cilantro

¼ cup chopped white onion

Green hot sauce

1. **Make the chili.** Heat the oil in a Dutch oven over medium-high heat. When the oil is hot, add the onion and cook, stirring occasionally, until starting to brown, about 7 minutes. Add the ground chicken, garlic, jalapeño, flour, cumin, and salt and sauté, breaking up the chicken as it cooks, until no longer pink. Stir in the sweet potato, broth, coconut milk, and chiles. Bring to a simmer, turn the heat to low, and simmer for 20 minutes, or until the sweet potato is tender.

2. **Garnish the dish and serve.** Season with salt. Serve the chili with your choice of garnishes.

Per Serving *(without garnishes): Calories: 319; Fat: 19g; Protein: 22g; Total Carbs: 17g; Fiber: 2g; Sodium: 926mg; Iron: 3mg*

Tandoori-Style Chicken Skewers with Cucumber Raita

Technically tandoori chicken is a marinated chicken dish cooked in a tandoor, a type of hot clay oven. In this case, it refers to the spiced yogurt marinade, but the skewers are cooked under a broiler. The marinade protects the chicken from high heat, keeping it tender. Cool, creamy cucumber raita makes a perfect accompaniment.

SERVES 4

Active time: 20 minutes
Total time: 20 minutes

....

LOW-CARB, NUT-FREE

FOR THE RAITA

½ cup plain coconut yogurt

2 teaspoons honey

2 tablespoons minced fresh mint

1 teaspoon sea salt

2 cups peeled, seeded, halved, and thinly sliced cucumber

Freshly ground black pepper

FOR THE CHICKEN

Olive or avocado oil spray, for greasing the pan

½ cup plain coconut yogurt

1 tablespoon freshly squeezed lemon juice

2 teaspoons minced garlic

2 teaspoons minced fresh ginger

2 teaspoons coconut sugar

2 teaspoons curry powder

1 teaspoon sea salt

1 pound boneless, skinless chicken thighs, cut into 1-inch pieces

1. **Get ready.** Arrange an oven rack 8 inches from the broiler element. Preheat the broiler. Line a rimmed baking sheet with aluminum foil and spray with oil.

2. **Make the raita.** In a small bowl, stir together the yogurt, honey, mint, and salt. Stir in the cucumber and toss to coat. Refrigerate until ready to serve.

3. **Prepare the chicken and serve.** In a large bowl, combine the yogurt, lemon juice, garlic, ginger, sugar, curry powder, and salt. Add the chicken and stir to coat. Thread the chicken loosely on 4 metal skewers. Arrange the skewers on the prepared baking sheet. Broil for 5 minutes, or until browned in spots. Turn the skewers and broil for another 5 minutes, or until the chicken is cooked through. Serve the skewers with the raita.

SERVING SUGGESTION: Offer a side dish of cauliflower rice seasoned with cumin.

Per Serving: Calories: 279; Fat: 13g; Protein: 30g; Total Carbs: 10g; Fiber: 1g; Sodium: 978mg; Iron: 2mg

Thai Basil Chicken with Green Beans

Thai basil is what gives this classic dish its signature flavor, but if you can't get your hands on it, you can substitute regular basil. This dish is meant to have the punch of heat, so don't skimp on the chiles.

SERVES 4

Active time: 25 minutes
Total time: 25 minutes

LOW-CARB, NUT-FREE

3 tablespoons maple syrup

2 tablespoons coconut aminos

2 tablespoons fish sauce

2 tablespoons avocado oil

1 or 2 Thai chiles or jalapeños, seeded (if desired) and minced

1 red bell pepper, seeded and chopped

8 ounces green beans, trimmed

1 pound ground chicken

4 scallions, white and green parts, cut into 1-inch pieces

3 garlic cloves, minced

1 cup thinly sliced fresh Thai basil or regular basil leaves

1. **Prepare the sauce.** In a small bowl, stir together the maple syrup, coconut aminos, and fish sauce. Set aside.

2. **Stir-fry the chicken and vegetables.** Heat the oil in a wok or 12-inch skillet over high heat. When the oil is hot, add the chiles and stir-fry for 1 minute. Add the bell pepper and green beans and stir-fry for 3 minutes. Add the chicken and use a spatula to break it up as it cooks. Add the scallions and garlic and stir-fry until the chicken is no longer pink. Stir in the basil and sauce and continue to cook until the sauce is reduced to a glaze, about 3 minutes. Serve.

SERVING SUGGESTIONS: In restaurants, this dish is served with a fried egg on top, so if you have the time, do it—it's incredibly delicious. Fry the eggs in avocado oil in the hot wok. You can also serve this dish with cauliflower rice.

Per Serving: Calories: 279; Fat: 13g; Protein: 30g; Total Carbs: 10g; Fiber: 1g; Sodium: 978mg; Iron: 2mg

Crispy Chicken Thighs with Roasted Apples, Onion, and Squash

Super crispy chicken thighs are one the easiest meals you can make, and they're incredibly tasty, too. Delicata squash is oblong with a yellow-and-green striped skin. You can eat the skin, which makes it really fast to prepare, and the flavor is subtly sweet. If you can't find it, substitute butternut squash.

SERVES 4

Prep time: 20 minutes
Cook time: 20 minutes

....
LOW-CARB, NUT-FREE

FOR THE VEGETABLES

2 pounds delicata squash, seeded and cut into ½-inch slices (about 3 cups)

2 apples, cored and cut into ½-inch slices

1 medium red onion, cut into ½-inch slices

1 tablespoon extra-virgin olive oil

Sea salt

FOR THE CHICKEN

4 bone-in, skin-on chicken thighs (about 1½ pounds)

Sea salt

1 tablespoon avocado oil

FOR THE SAUCE

1½ cups fresh cilantro leaves

2 scallions, white and green parts, chopped

1 tablespoon minced jalapeño

1 tablespoon freshly squeezed lemon juice

⅓ cup extra-virgin olive oil

½ teaspoon sea salt

Freshly ground black pepper

1. **Get ready.** Preheat the oven to 425°F. Line a rimmed baking sheet with parchment paper or aluminum foil.

2. **Make the vegetables.** In a large bowl, combine the squash, apples, onion, olive oil, and a pinch of salt and toss to coat. Spread the vegetables evenly on the prepared baking sheet. Roast for 15 to 20 minutes, until the vegetables are lightly browned.

3. **Prepare the chicken.** Meanwhile, using kitchen shears or a sharp knife, carefully remove the bones from chicken thighs, leaving the skin intact. (Freeze the bones to use when making Rich Chicken Broth, page 158.) Pat the chicken dry with paper towels and season both sides generously with salt.

4. **Cook the chicken.** Heat the oil in a 12-inch skillet over medium heat. When the oil is hot, add the chicken thighs, skin-side down, to the pan. Cook the chicken, without turning, until deeply golden brown and crisp, 10 minutes. Don't rush the process—if the thighs are spattering a lot and getting brown too fast, turn the heat down a bit. You want them to be sizzling and slowly browning, not flash-frying. Flip the thighs and finish cooking through, 3 to 5 more minutes. Transfer to a cutting board and let them rest for 5 minutes, then cut into ¾-inch slices.

5. **Make the sauce.** While the chicken cooks, combine the cilantro, scallions, jalapeño, lemon juice, olive oil, salt, and pepper in a food processor and pulse to make a chunky pesto. Taste and add more salt as needed.

6. **Assemble and serve.** Divide the chicken and vegetables among four plates. Top with the sauce and serve.

SMART SHOPPING: To save time, ask your butcher to remove the chicken bones.

Per Serving: *Calories: 363; Fat: 75g; Protein: 13g; Total Carbs: 19g; Fiber: 4g; Sodium: 360mg; Iron: 2mg*

Turkey Tenderloin with Raw Cranberry Salsa and Smashed Potatoes

Think of this dish as a weeknight twist on Thanksgiving. The turkey tenderloins are pounded thin so they cook quickly, then coated in chopped pecans and coconut and baked for a crispy finish. I love the raw cranberry salsa with turkey, but it's great with tortilla chips, too.

SERVES 4

Active time: 30 minutes
Total time: 30 minutes

FOR THE POTATOES

1 pound small new potatoes, halved or quartered

3 tablespoons ghee or extra-virgin olive oil

⅓ cup almond milk

2 tablespoons thinly sliced scallions, green parts only

Freshly ground black pepper

Sea salt

FOR THE TURKEY

1 (1-pound) turkey tenderloin, cut into 4 equal pieces

1½ cups pecans

¼ cup unsweetened shredded coconut

1 teaspoon sea salt

Freshly ground black pepper

1 large egg

FOR THE SALSA

1 (12-ounce) bag fresh cranberries

½ cup chopped fresh cilantro

3 scallions, white and green parts, chopped

1 jalapeño, seeded (if desired) and chopped

Juice of 1 lime

½ cup coconut sugar

½ teaspoon sea salt

1. **Get ready.** Preheat the oven to 400°F. Line a rimmed baking sheet with parchment paper or aluminum foil.

2. **Make the potatoes.** Fill a large pot with cold, salted water. Add the potatoes and bring to a boil over medium-high heat. Lower the heat and simmer the potatoes until tender, 10 to 15 minutes. Drain the potatoes and return them to the pot. Add the ghee and use a potato masher to coarsely mash the potatoes. Stir in the almond milk, scallions, and several grinds of pepper. Season with salt as needed. Keep warm.

3. **Prepare the turkey.** While the potatoes cook, place each piece of turkey between sheets of plastic wrap and use a meat mallet or rolling pin to pound into cutlets about ½ inch thick. Combine the pecans, coconut, salt, and several grinds of pepper in a food processor. Pulse until the mixture is the texture of coarse sand (do not purée into a paste). Scrape the mixture out onto a large plate (rinse and dry the food processor bowl). In a pie plate or shallow dish, beat the egg. One at a time, dip the turkey cutlets into the egg, shaking off the excess, then transfer to the chopped pecan mixture. Press the cutlets into the mixture, then flip over to coat the other side. Transfer to the prepared baking sheet. Bake for 10 minutes,

flip the tenderloins with a spatula, and bake for another 10 minutes, or until nicely crispy.

4. **Make the salsa.** While the turkey bakes, combine the cranberries, cilantro, scallions, jalapeño, lime juice, sugar, and salt in the food processor and chop to a chunky purée (do not blend until smooth). Taste and add more sugar and/or salt as needed. Scrape into a bowl.

5. **Assemble and serve.** Divide the potatoes and turkey among four dinner plates. Season the turkey with salt, then add a few spoonfuls of salsa and a few grinds of black pepper. Serve.

Per Serving: *Calories: 603; Fat: 31g; Protein: 41g; Total Carbs: 43g; Fiber: 8g; Sodium: 998mg; Iron: 3mg*

Chicken and Dumplings

When I first started hosting dinner parties in my twenties, my signature dish was chicken and dumplings. I'd start with a whole chicken in the pot and spend hours making the broth, straining it, then cooking vegetables and finally the dumplings. Over time, I streamlined the process for weeknight dinners. Make sure to keep the dumplings small so they cook quickly.

SERVES 4

Active time: 30 minutes
Total time: 30 minutes

. . . .
LOW-CARB, ONE-PAN

FOR THE SOUP

3 tablespoons ghee or avocado oil

1 cup peeled and diced carrot

1 cup finely chopped yellow onion

1 garlic clove, minced

1 teaspoon dried thyme

1 teaspoon sea salt

¼ teaspoon nutmeg

1 tablespoon cassava flour

1 pound boneless, skinless chicken thighs

4 cups Rich Chicken Broth (page 158) or store-bought chicken broth

FOR THE DUMPLINGS

¾ cup almond flour

¾ cup cassava flour

2 teaspoons baking powder

½ teaspoon dried thyme

1 teaspoon sea salt

½ cup canned full-fat coconut milk

1 large egg, lightly beaten

FOR FINISHING

½ cup canned full-fat coconut milk

Sea salt

Freshly ground black pepper

1. **Prepare the soup.** Heat the ghee in a Dutch oven or casserole with a tight-fitting lid over medium-high heat. When the ghee is hot, add the carrot, onion, garlic, thyme, salt, and nutmeg and sauté the vegetables, stirring occasionally, for 5 minutes. Add the flour and sauté for another 5 minutes. Add the chicken thighs and broth and bring to a boil. Turn down the heat to medium-low so the broth is just simmering. Partially cover and simmer for 15 minutes.

2. **Make the dumplings.** While the soup is simmering, in a medium bowl, stir together the almond flour, cassava flour, baking powder, thyme, salt, coconut milk, and egg until well combined. Roll the batter into ½-inch balls. Add the dumplings to the gently simmering soup, cover, and cook for 5 minutes.

3. **Finish the soup.** Remove the chicken thighs and use two forks to pull the meat into bite-size pieces. Return the chicken to pot. Stir in the coconut milk, then season with salt and pepper. Serve.

SMART SHOPPING: To streamline the process even more, use rotisserie chicken.

Per Serving: *Calories: 694; Fat: 47g; Protein: 40g; Total Carbs: 30g; Fiber: 4g; Sodium: 947mg; Iron: 4mg*

Curried Chicken Meatball Bowls

This is in effect a warm-cool salad, with crunchy slaw topped with warm meatballs and a generous drizzle of creamy tahini sauce. These meatballs freeze really well, so consider doubling the batch and freezing half. Notice that there's chopped cilantro as well as freshly squeezed lemon juice in more than one place, so that you can streamline your prep.

SERVES 4

Active time: 25 minutes
Total time: 25 minutes

....
LOW-CARB

FOR THE MEATBALLS

1 pound ground chicken

¼ medium yellow onion, grated

¼ cup finely chopped fresh parsley

¼ cup finely chopped fresh cilantro

2 teaspoons honey

1 tablespoon arrowroot starch

2 teaspoons curry powder

½ teaspoon smoked paprika

1 teaspoon sea salt

FOR THE SAUCE

½ cup tahini

¼ cup freshly squeezed lemon juice

½ teaspoon sea salt

¼ teaspoon curry powder

FOR THE SLAW

4 cups shredded cabbage

4 tablespoons raisins

4 tablespoons chopped
toasted almonds

2 tablespoons chopped Pickled Red
Onions (page 165)

¼ cup finely chopped fresh cilantro

1 tablespoon freshly squeezed
lemon juice

Sea salt

1. **Get ready.** Preheat the oven to 400°F. Line a rimmed baking sheet with parchment paper or aluminum foil.

2. **Make the meatballs.** In a large bowl, combine the chicken, onion, parsley, cilantro, honey, arrowroot, curry powder, paprika, and salt and mix together with your hands. Ground chicken can be sticky to work with; coating your hands with a few drops of olive oil will make shaping the meatballs go much more smoothly. Form 1-inch meatballs and set them on the prepared baking sheet. Bake the meatballs for 20 minutes, or until lightly browned and cooked through.

3. **Make the sauce.** Meanwhile, in a medium bowl, stir together the tahini, lemon juice, salt, and curry powder.

Stir in water, a tablespoon at a time (the mixture will seize up, but keep stirring), until the sauce is the consistency of thick cream. Taste and add more salt as needed.

4. **Make the slaw.** In a medium bowl, combine the cabbage, raisins, almonds, pickled onions, cilantro, lemon juice, and salt and toss to combine.

5. **Assemble the bowls.** Divide the slaw among four shallow bowls and top with the meatballs. Drizzle with the sauce and serve.

SMART SHOPPING: Purchase coleslaw mix to save time shredding cabbage.

Per Serving: *Calories: 368; Fat: 22g; Protein: 27g; Total Carbs: 20g; Fiber: 6g; Sodium: 998mg; Iron: 4mg*

Pan-Roasted Chicken with Figs and Mushrooms

My grocery store doesn't sell boneless, skin-on chicken breasts, so I ask the butcher to bone skin-on breasts for me. The chicken breasts cook much more quickly without bones, and preparing the dish with skinless chicken breasts wouldn't be nearly as tasty.

SERVES 4

Active time: 30 minutes
Total time: 30 minutes

. . . .

LOW-CARB, NUT-FREE

4 boneless, skin-on chicken breast halves (about 1 pound)

Sea salt

4 tablespoons avocado oil, divided

2 shallots, minced

2 cups quartered ripe figs

2 cups quartered button mushrooms

1 teaspoon minced fresh thyme

Juice of ½ lemon

1. **Make the chicken.** Season the chicken on both sides with salt. Heat 2 tablespoons of oil in a 12- or 14-inch oven-safe skillet over medium-high heat. When the oil is very hot, add the chicken breasts, skin-side down. Cook the chicken without moving until the skin is golden brown, 7 to 8 minutes. Flip the chicken and cook for 5 minutes, or until just cooked through. Transfer to a cutting board to rest.

2. **Make the mushrooms.** Return the same pan to medium heat and add the remaining 2 tablespoons of oil. Add the shallot and sauté, scraping up the browned bits and juices, until translucent, about 3 minutes. Add the mushrooms and a pinch of salt and sauté until browned and tender, about 5 minutes. Transfer the mixture to a medium bowl and keep warm.

3. **Make the figs.** Return the pan to medium heat and add the figs, cut-side down. Let the figs cook, without stirring, for 3 minutes. Add the figs to the bowl with the mushrooms. Add the thyme and a squeeze of the lemon and toss to combine. Season with salt.

4. **Serve.** Slice the chicken and divide among four plates. Divide the figs and mushrooms among the plates and serve.

SERVING SUGGESTION: Cashew Cheese (see page 163), especially made with chives and tarragon, would be a lovely, creamy accompaniment.

Per Serving: *Calories: 463; Fat: 28g; Protein: 33g; Total Carbs: 22g; Fiber: 4g; Sodium: 672mg; Iron: 2mg*

Chicken Fajita Salad

Raise your hand if you were obsessed with fajitas in the 1980s and 1990s (my hand is raised). The whole ritual was so fun, with sizzling platters of meat and vegetables whisked to your table, along with warm tortillas and all the fixings. This salad is a lighter, healthier, one-pan take on those vibrant days, but with all the nostalgic flavor.

SERVES 4

Active time: 30 minutes
Total time: 30 minutes

....

LOW-CARB, NUT-FREE, ONE-PAN

FOR THE VEGETABLES

2 green bell peppers, seeded and cut into ½-inch strips

1 medium red onion, cut into ½-inch slices

½ lime, halved

1 tablespoon avocado oil

1 teaspoon chili powder

½ teaspoon sea salt

FOR THE DRESSING

1 cup fresh cilantro leaves

1 jalapeño, seeded and finely chopped

¼ cup plain coconut yogurt

1 garlic clove, chopped

1½ tablespoons freshly squeezed lime juice

¾ teaspoon sea salt

½ cup extra-virgin olive oil

FOR THE CHICKEN

1 pound boneless, skinless chicken breast halves, cut into ¼-inch strips

1 tablespoon avocado oil

1 teaspoon chili powder

1 teaspoon dried oregano

½ teaspoon sea salt

FOR THE SALAD

4 cups salad greens

1. **Get ready.** Arrange an oven rack 6 inches from the broiler element and another oven rack in center of the oven. Preheat the oven to 425°F. Line a rimmed baking sheet with aluminum foil.

2. **Roast the vegetables.** In a large bowl, toss the bell peppers, onion, and lime wedges with the oil, chili powder, and salt. Spread the vegetables on the prepared baking sheet (reserve the bowl). Roast for 10 minutes. Remove the pan from oven and turn on the broiler.

3. **Prepare the dressing.** Meanwhile, combine the cilantro, jalapeño, yogurt, garlic, lime juice, salt and olive oil in a blender and purée until smooth. Taste and add more salt as needed.

Continued >

4. **Broil the chicken and vegetables.** In a large bowl, toss the chicken with the oil, chili powder, oregano, and salt. When the vegetables are done, add the chicken to the pan, nestling the slices among the vegetables. Broil the chicken and vegetables for 5 minutes, or until the chicken is cooked through (watch carefully) and vegetables are browning in spots. Remove from the oven and squeeze the roasted lime wedges over the chicken and vegetables.

5. **Assemble the salad and serve.** Divide the salad greens among four shallow bowls. Top with the chicken and vegetables. Spoon the dressing over the salads and serve warm.

SERVING SUGGESTION: Big dollops of guacamole would be fantastic atop the salads.

Per Serving: *Calories: 344; Fat: 23g; Protein: 28g; Total Carbs: 6g; Fiber: 1g; Sodium: 884mg; Iron: 2mg*

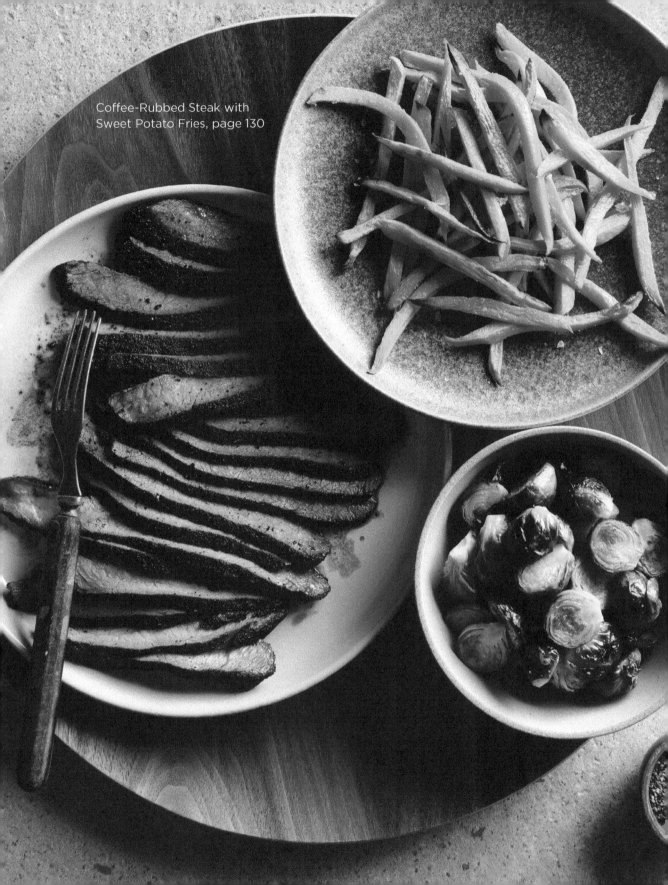

Coffee-Rubbed Steak with
Sweet Potato Fries, page 130

CHAPTER SEVEN

Beef, Pork, and Lamb

Greek Meatza with Yogurt Sauce

I think of meatza as a cross between a burger and pizza. In this case, a seasoned meat base is topped with Greek salad and drizzled with green yogurt sauce. Keep this meatza base recipe on hand and change up the toppings depending on what you have or what you're craving. Store leftover yogurt sauce in a glass jar in the refrigerator—it's a great sauce for dipping vegetables.

SERVES 4

Active time: 20 minutes
Total time: 25 minutes

....

LOW-CARB, NUT-FREE

FOR THE MEATZA

1 pound ground beef

½ medium yellow onion, minced

2 garlic cloves, minced

2 teaspoons arrowroot starch

1 teaspoon dried oregano

1 teaspoon sea salt

Freshly ground black pepper

FOR THE YOGURT SAUCE

1 cup plain coconut yogurt

½ cup chopped fresh parsley leaves

¼ cup chopped fresh dill

2 garlic cloves, minced

1 teaspoon sea salt

Freshly ground black pepper

FOR FINISHING

2 cups torn romaine lettuce leaves

12 cherry tomatoes, chopped

½ cup cucumber, cut into ½-inch pieces

12 kalamata olives, pitted and chopped

4 pepperoncini, cut into ¼-inch slices

2 tablespoons chopped Pickled Red Onions (page 165)

2 tablespoons chopped fresh dill

Sea salt

Freshly ground black pepper

1. **Get ready.** Preheat the oven to 400°F. Line a rimmed baking sheet with parchment paper or aluminum foil.

2. **Prepare the meatza.** In a large bowl, combine the beef, onion, garlic, arrow-root, oregano, salt, and several grinds of pepper. Using your hands, mix gently until thoroughly combined. Transfer the meat to the prepared pan and pat the meatza out into a ¼-inch-thick oblong patty. Bake for 20 minutes.

3. **Make the yogurt sauce.** Meanwhile, combine the yogurt, parsley, dill, garlic, salt, and pepper in a blender and blend until smooth.

4. **Finish the meatza and serve.** Top the meatza with the romaine, tomatoes, cucumber, olives, pepperoncini, pickled onions, and dill. Drizzle with the yogurt sauce. Season with salt and pepper, cut into squares, and serve.

SERVING SUGGESTION: Crisp roasted potatoes taste great alongside this meatza. Dip them in the yogurt sauce!

SIMPLE SWAP: Substitute ground lamb or ground pork for half of the ground beef.

Per Serving: *Calories: 373; Fat: 20g; Protein: 35g; Total Carbs: 16g; Fiber: 3g; Sodium: 1,105mg; Iron: 5mg*

Vietnamese Pork in Lettuce Wraps

With plenty of whole fresh mint and cilantro leaves rolled up with the lettuce, I can't believe it took me so long to realize how delicious lettuce wraps are. The bright, fresh flavors are the perfect complement to sizzling hot pork. You'll need a dozen 3-inch-long wooden skewers for these.

SERVE 4

Active time: 20 minutes
Total time: 25 minutes

....
LOW-CARB, NUT-FREE

FOR THE SKEWERS

1 pound ground pork

3 tablespoons fish sauce

1 tablespoon honey

½ jalapeño, seeded (if desired) and minced

2 scallions, white and green parts, minced

1 large garlic clove, minced

FOR THE DIPPING SAUCE

3 tablespoons freshly squeezed lime juice

1½ tablespoons toasted sesame oil

1 tablespoon honey

1 tablespoon coconut aminos

1 tablespoon fish sauce

2 teaspoons grated fresh ginger

1 garlic clove, minced

FOR THE LETTUCE WRAPS

1 head butter lettuce, separated into leaves

1 cup thinly sliced radishes

1 cup fresh mint leaves

1 cup fresh cilantro leaves

1 lime, cut into wedges, for garnish

1. **Get ready.** Arrange an oven rack about 8 inches from the broiler element. Preheat the broiler. Line a rimmed baking sheet with aluminum foil.

2. **Make the skewers.** Combine the pork, fish sauce, honey, jalapeño, scallions, and garlic in a large bowl. Using your hands, gently mix the seasonings into the pork. Press about 2 tablespoons of the pork mixture around each skewer, forming a cigar shape and leaving a bit of empty skewer at each end. Place the skewers on the prepared baking sheet. Broil, turning once, until nicely browned, 6 to 8 minutes total (watch them carefully).

3. **Make the dipping sauce.** Stir together the lime juice, sesame oil, honey, coconut aminos, fish sauce, ginger, and garlic in a small bowl. Taste and adjust the seasoning as needed.

4. **Prepare the lettuce wraps and serve.**
   Push the pork off each skewer and
   divide among four dinner plates.
   Serve hot, rolled in the lettuce leaves
   with the radishes, mint, cilantro,
   dipping sauce, and lime wedges
   for squeezing.

SERVING SUGGESTION: Serve the wraps
with cauliflower rice.

Per Serving: *Calories: 448; Fat: 29g; Protein: 31g;
Total Carbs: 16g; Fiber: 3g; Sodium: 998mg;
Iron: 2mg*

Coffee-Rubbed Steak with Sweet Potato Fries

In this recipe, a simple rub adds an incredible amount of spicy-smoky flavor to steak. The trick for crispy sweet potato fries is to cut them into thin steaks, preheat the pan, and roast them in the top third of the oven. Sweet potato fries can go from almost done to burned very quickly, so keep a careful eye on them.

SERVES 4

Active time: 25 minutes
Total time: 30 minutes

....

LOW-CARB, NUT-FREE

FOR THE FRIES

1 pound sweet potatoes, peeled and cut into ¼-inch-thick fries

1 tablespoon avocado oil

½ teaspoon garlic powder

1 teaspoon salt

Freshly ground black pepper

FOR THE STEAK

¼ cup freshly ground coffee grounds (you can use decaf, but do not use instant coffee granules)

4 teaspoons coconut sugar

2 teaspoons chili powder

2 teaspoons ground cumin

2 teaspoons sea salt

Freshly ground black pepper

1 (1-pound) flatiron or skirt steak

1 tablespoon avocado oil

1 lime, cut into wedges, for garnish

1. **Get ready.** Arrange an oven rack in the top third of the oven. Preheat the oven to 400°F. Line a rimmed baking sheet with parchment paper or aluminum foil and put the baking sheet in the oven to preheat as well.

2. **Make the fries.** In a large bowl, toss the potatoes with the oil, garlic powder, salt, and a few grinds of pepper. Remove the baking sheet from the oven and spread out the potatoes evenly on it. Place the sheet on the higher oven rack and roast for 10 minutes. Turn the potatoes and roast for another 5 to 10 minutes, until crisp. Watch carefully so they don't burn.

3. **Make the steak.** Meanwhile, in a small bowl, combine the coffee grounds, sugar, chili powder, cumin, salt, and a few grinds of pepper. Sprinkle generously all over the steak and rub it in. Set a 12-inch cast iron skillet over medium-high heat. When the pan is hot, add the oil and tilt to spread it evenly over the pan. Add the

steak and sear for 4 minutes. Flip the steak and sear for another 4 minutes. Continue searing and flipping until the steak reaches your desired doneness. (For medium, the meat should feel springy, not squishy, when poked.) Transfer the steak to a cutting board and let rest for 5 minutes.

4. **Serve.** Divide the fries among four dinner plates. Slice the steak thinly against the grain and serve with squeezes of lime and additional salt.

SIMPLE SWAP: You can make the fries with Yukon Gold potatoes; just add a few more minutes of roasting time.

SERVING SUGGESTION: Roast Brussels sprouts on a second baking sheet to serve with the steak and fries.

Per Serving: *Calories: 355; Fat: 17g; Protein: 25g; Total Carbs: 28g; Fiber: 3g; Sodium: 1,214mg; Iron: 4mg*

Souvlaki with Cucumber Sauce and Greek Salad

I love sauces where you just dump everything into a blender and purée until smooth—small effort, big flavor! Using the sauce for both the salad and souvlaki saves you from having to make a separate salad dressing. If you have extra cucumber, chop it up and add it to the salad.

SERVES 4

Active time: 25 minutes
Total time: 30 minutes

....

LOW-CARB, NUT-FREE

FOR THE SAUCE

1 cup plain coconut yogurt

¼ cup fresh mint leaves

¼ cup fresh dill

¼ cup chopped, peeled cucumber

2 garlic cloves, chopped

2 tablespoons extra-virgin olive oil

1 teaspoon sea salt

Freshly ground black pepper

FOR THE SOUVLAKI

¼ cup freshly squeezed lemon juice

3 tablespoons extra-virgin olive oil

4 garlic cloves, minced

1 tablespoon dried oregano

1 teaspoon red pepper flakes

½ teaspoon sea salt

Freshly ground black pepper

1 (1-pound) pork tenderloin, cut into 1-inch pieces

FOR THE SALAD

4 cups torn romaine leaves

2 tablespoons chopped scallions, white and green parts

2 tablespoons chopped fresh dill

8 kalamata olives, pitted and halved

Freshly ground black pepper

1. **Get ready.** Arrange an oven rack 8 inches from the broiler element. Preheat the broiler. Line a rimmed baking sheet with aluminum foil.

2. **Make the sauce.** Combine the yogurt, mint, dill, cucumber, garlic, olive oil, salt, and pepper in a blender or food processor and blend until smooth. Transfer to a jar and refrigerate while you make the souvlaki.

3. **Make the souvlaki.** In a large bowl, combine the lemon juice, olive oil, garlic, oregano, red pepper flakes, salt, black pepper, and pork and toss to coat the pork thoroughly. Thread the pork loosely on metal or wooden skewers and place them on the prepared baking sheet. Broil for 4 minutes per

side, or until just cooked through. Let rest for 5 minutes.

4. **Make the salad and serve.** In a medium bowl, toss together the romaine, scallions, dill, and olives. Divide the salad among four dinner plates. Add the skewers to the plates. Top the salad and skewers with cucumber sauce and a few grinds of pepper and serve.

COOKING HACK: You can also grill these skewers over high heat for 4 to 6 minutes per side.

SERVING SUGGESTION: If you have time, fill out the salad with sliced radishes, red bell pepper, tomato, and/or pepperoncini.

Per Serving: *Calories: 355; Fat: 20g; Protein: 35g; Total Carbs: 9g; Fiber: 1g; Sodium: 1,124mg; Iron: 3mg*

Kid-Friendly Meat Sauce with Spaghetti Squash

When my son was young, he preferred spaghetti with smooth sauce, so I started making meat sauce with tomato sauce instead of chopped tomatoes. It has the bonus of coming together more quickly as well, because you don't have to simmer the sauce long enough to break down the tomatoes. Microwaving spaghetti squash instead of roasting it cuts the cooking time down to 15 minutes. If you like, save the squash seeds and roast them for a snack.

SERVES 4

Active time: 25 minutes
Total time: 30 minutes

....

LOW-CARB, NUT-FREE

FOR THE SAUCE

1 tablespoon extra-virgin olive oil

½ cup minced yellow onion

2 garlic cloves, minced

8 ounces ground beef

8 ounces sweet Italian sausage

1 (28-ounce) can tomato sauce

1 teaspoon coconut sugar

1 tablespoon dried Italian
    seasoning blend

½ teaspoon sea salt

FOR THE SPAGHETTI SQUASH

1 (3- to 4-pound) spaghetti squash,
    halved lengthwise and seeded

2 teaspoons extra-virgin olive oil

1 teaspoon garlic powder

Sea salt

1. **Make the sauce.** Heat the oil in a Dutch oven over medium-high heat. When the oil is hot, add the onion and sauté, stirring occasionally, until softened, about 5 minutes. Add the garlic, beef, and sausage and sauté, breaking up the meat with a spoon, until the meat is just cooked through, about 7 minutes. Add the tomato sauce, sugar, Italian seasoning, and salt. Simmer for 15 minutes, stirring occasionally. Season with more salt as needed.

2. **Make the spaghetti squash and serve.** Meanwhile, pour ¼ inch of water into a glass 9-by-13-inch baking dish. Rub the oil into the flesh-side of each squash half, then season with the garlic powder and salt. Put the squash halves, cut-side down, in the dish. Microwave on high for 10 to 15 minutes, until tender. Use a fork to pull the squash into strands. Divide the squash among four shallow bowls. Top with the meat sauce and serve.

COOKING HACK: If you can't fit a large baking dish in your microwave, microwave each squash half separately in a smaller dish.

Per Serving: *Calories: 381; Fat: 20g; Protein: 27g; Total Carbs: 25g; Fiber: 6g; Sodium: 703mg; Iron: 5mg*

Lamb Chops with Gremolata, New Potatoes, and Green Beans

Gremolata is a hand-chopped pesto made with lemon zest and parsley. It's very bright and fresh, which makes it a perfect accompaniment to rich meats. (It's traditionally served with osso buco, the famous Italian dish of braised veal shanks.) I started pairing it with rich lamb chops years ago, and it quickly became my family's favorite way to enjoy lamb. It also happens to taste amazing with potatoes and green beans.

SERVES 4

Active time: 20 minutes
Total time: 30 minutes

....
LOW-CARB, NUT-FREE

FOR THE POTATOES AND GREEN BEANS

1 pound 1-inch new potatoes

4 cups trimmed green beans

2 tablespoons ghee or extra-virgin olive oil

1 tablespoon freshly squeezed lemon juice

Sea salt

FOR THE LAMB CHOPS

1 (8-rib) rack of lamb, cut into 4 (2-rib) sections

Sea salt

FOR THE GREMOLATA

Grated zest of 2 lemons

½ cup fresh parsley leaves

4 garlic cloves, halved

¼ teaspoon sea salt

1 teaspoon extra-virgin olive oil

1. **Get ready.** Preheat the grill for indirect heat: With a gas grill, leave a couple of the burners on high and turn one off. With charcoal, push the embers off to one side.

2. **Make the potatoes and green beans.** Fill a large pot with cold, salted water and add the potatoes. Bring the water to a boil over high heat, then reduce the heat to medium-high. Add the green beans and bring the water back to a boil. Cook the potatoes and green beans together until both are just tender, about 5 minutes. Drain the potatoes and green beans, then return them to the pot. Add the ghee and lemon juice to the pot and stir to coat the vegetables. Season with salt. Keep warm.

3. **Make the lamb chops.** Sprinkle the lamb all over with salt. Grill the chops over indirect heat (to prevent flare-ups from dripping fat), about

4½ minutes per side for medium (pink, not red). Transfer the chops to a cutting board and let rest for 10 minutes, then cut each section in half.

4. **Make the gremolata.** While the lamb rests, combine the lemon zest, parsley, garlic, and salt on a cutting board. Using a chef's knife, mince the ingredients together into a coarse pesto.

Scrape into a bowl and stir in the olive oil.

5. **Assemble and serve.** Divide the lamb, potatoes, and green beans among four plates. Top the lamb with gremolata and serve immediately.

Per Serving: *Calories: 313; Fat: 12g; Protein: 27g; Total Carbs: 27g; Fiber: 5g; Sodium: 316mg; Iron: 4mg*

Lamb-Stuffed Zucchini Boats

Crunchy pine nuts and fragrant lamb nestled into tender zucchini boats make for a simple, flavorful, and pretty dinner. I love these drizzled with a simple tahini sauce, but you could also top them with your favorite yogurt sauce or tomato sauce.

SERVES 4

Active time: 30 minutes
Total time: 30 minutes

....
LOW-CARB

FOR THE ZUCCHINI

4 (6-inch) zucchini

Sea salt

FOR THE LAMB FILLING

1 tablespoon extra-virgin olive oil

¼ cup pine nuts

½ medium yellow onion,
   finely chopped

3 garlic cloves, minced

1 pound ground lamb

1 tablespoon dried oregano

¼ teaspoon ground nutmeg

1 teaspoon sea salt

Freshly ground black pepper

2 cups coarsely chopped spinach
   leaves, stems removed

2 teaspoons arrowroot starch

FOR THE SAUCE

½ cup tahini

¼ cup freshly squeezed lemon juice

½ teaspoon ground cumin

½ teaspoon sea salt

1. **Get ready.** Preheat the oven to 425°F. Line a rimmed baking sheet with parchment paper or aluminum foil.

2. **Prepare the zucchini.** Halve each zucchini lengthwise. Using a spoon, scoop out the seeds and some of the flesh to create "boats." Season the cut sides with salt, then put the zucchini, cut-side down, on the prepared baking sheet. Bake for 15 minutes.

3. **Prepare the lamb filling.** Meanwhile, heat the oil in a 12-inch skillet over medium heat. When the oil is hot, add the pine nuts and cook, stirring constantly, until the nuts are toasted, about 3 minutes. Using a slotted spoon, transfer the nuts to a plate. Add the onion to the same pan and sauté until it begins to soften, about 5 minutes. Stir in the garlic, lamb, oregano, nutmeg, salt, and several grinds of pepper and sauté, breaking up the lamb with the spatula, until the meat is no longer pink, about 7 minutes. Stir in the spinach and sauté until wilted, about 3 minutes. Stir in the arrowroot and toasted pine nuts and sauté for 1 minute. Remove the pan from the heat.

4. **Bake the zucchini boats.** Turn the zucchini boats over and divide the lamb filling among them. Bake for 10 minutes.

5. **Make the sauce.** While the boats bake, in a medium bowl, stir together the tahini, lemon juice, cumin, and salt. Stir in water, a tablespoon at a time (the mixture will seize up, but keep stirring), until the sauce is the consistency of thick cream. Taste and add more salt as needed.

6. **Serve.** Place 2 boats on each of four dinner plates, drizzle with sauce, and serve.

SERVING SUGGESTION: Roasted new potatoes tossed with extra-virgin olive oil, garlic, and dill would be amazing on the side—simply roast them on a separate baking sheet while the zucchini boats bake.

Per Serving: *Calories: 313; Fat: 12g; Protein: 27g; Total Carbs: 27g; Fiber: 5g; Sodium: 316mg; Iron: 4mg*

Orange Beef and Broccoli

Orange beef is my son's favorite Chinese take-out dish. This is a lighter version—no breading, less sugar—but still tastes fantastic. I think beef and broccoli is one of the world's great meat and vegetable combinations, especially when the broccoli is tender-crisp. If you don't have a wok, use a 12-inch skillet.

SERVES 4

Active time: 20 minutes
Total time: 20 minutes

LOW-CARB, NUT-FREE

FOR THE SAUCE

Grated zest of 1 orange

½ cup freshly squeezed orange juice

¼ cup coconut aminos

2 tablespoons maple syrup

1½ tablespoons apple cider vinegar

1 tablespoon fish sauce

4 garlic cloves, minced

1 (2-inch) piece fresh ginger, peeled and minced

FOR THE BROCCOLI

1 tablespoon avocado oil

4 cups broccoli florets (from about 2 heads of broccoli)

2 tablespoons water

FOR THE STEAK

¼ cup arrowroot starch

1 teaspoon sea salt

1 (1-pound) flank steak, cut across the grain into ¼-inch slices

2 tablespoons avocado oil

¼ cup sliced scallions, white and green parts, for garnish

1. **Prepare the sauce.** In a small bowl, stir together the orange zest and juice, coconut aminos, maple syrup, vinegar, fish sauce, garlic, and ginger. Set aside.

2. **Stir-fry the broccoli.** Heat 1 tablespoon of oil in a wok over high heat. When the oil is hot, add the broccoli and stir-fry until the broccoli is browning at the edges, about 3 minutes. Add the water and continue to stir-fry until the water is evaporated and the broccoli is tender-crisp. Transfer the broccoli to a large bowl.

3. **Prepare the steak.** Combine the arrowroot and salt in a large zip-top bag. Add the steak, seal the bag, and toss to coat. Return the wok to high heat and add 1 tablespoon of oil. When the oil is hot, add the coated steak in batches and stir-fry until the steak is lightly browned, 2 to 3 minutes per side. Use the remaining 1 tablespoon of oil as needed. Transfer the steak to the bowl of broccoli as you go.

4. **Finish the dish.** Return the steak and broccoli to the wok. Pour in the sauce and bring to a simmer. Toss the steak and broccoli until the sauce is a glaze, about 3 minutes. Divide the steak and broccoli among four bowls. Top with the scallions and serve.

SERVING SUGGESTION: Cauliflower rice would make a terrific side.

Per Serving: *Calories: 364; Fat: 17g; Protein: 30g; Total Carbs: 25g; Fiber: 3g; Sodium: 1,178mg; Iron: 3mg*

Pan-Seared Steak with Creamed Mushrooms and Spinach

This is a classic steakhouse dish—not exactly light, but most definitely a treat. And it's an easy treat to boot, as everything cooks in one pan. If you have time, add baked potatoes (even microwaved baked potatoes!) with a pat of ghee and a sprinkle of minced chives.

SERVES 4

Active time: 20 minutes
Total time: 20 minutes

....

LOW-CARB, NUT-FREE, ONE-PAN

1 (1-pound) boneless ribeye or New York strip steak

Sea salt

1 tablespoon avocado oil

4 tablespoons ghee or extra-virgin olive oil, divided

3 ounces button mushrooms, quartered

2 garlic cloves, thinly sliced

6 cups coarsely chopped spinach leaves, stems removed

½ cup coconut cream

Freshly ground black pepper

1. **Sear the steak.** Pat the steak dry with a paper towel and season it with salt all over. Set a 12-inch cast iron skillet over medium-high heat. When the pan is very hot, add the oil and tilt the pan to spread it evenly. Add the steak and cook for 4 minutes. Flip the steak and cook to your desired doneness,
another 3 to 4 minutes. Transfer the steak to a cutting board and let rest.

2. **Make the mushrooms and spinach.** Add 2 tablespoons of ghee to the same pan. When the oil is hot, add the mushrooms and a generous pinch of salt. Sauté the mushrooms, stirring occasionally, until nicely browned, about 8 minutes. Add the remaining 2 tablespoons of ghee, the garlic, and spinach to the pan and sauté until the spinach is wilted, about 5 minutes. Transfer the spinach and mushrooms to a bowl and drain off any water from the pan. Return the pan to the heat and add the coconut cream and a pinch of salt. Bring to a simmer, stirring frequently. Pour the hot cream over the spinach mixture and toss to coat. Season with salt and pepper.

3. **Serve.** Slice the steak against the grain and divide among four dinner plates. Divide the spinach and mushrooms among the plates and serve.

SMART SHOPPING: Coconut cream can be purchased on its own, or you can use the solid cream at the top of a can of full-fat coconut milk.

COOKING HACK: For perfectly cooked steak, insert an instant-read thermometer into the center of the steak. Medium-rare is 135°F, and medium is 145°F.

Per Serving: *Calories: 405; Fat: 26g; Protein: 36g; Total Carbs: 12g; Fiber: 7g; Sodium: 574mg; Iron: 7mg*

Salisbury Steaks with Mushroom Gravy and Spinach Salad

As a kid, when my parents went out for dinner, our babysitter would make my sister and me Salisbury steak TV dinners. I loved those nights, so for me Salisbury steaks are wrapped up with nostalgia and fun memories. The TV dinner version probably wasn't all that delicious, but this scratch version totally is, with tender meat, caramelized onions, and rich mushroom gravy.

SERVES 4

Active time: 30 minutes
Total time: 30 minutes
....
LOW-CARB, NUT-FREE

FOR THE STEAKS AND GRAVY

8 ounces ground beef

8 ounces ground pork

½ cup Caramelized Onions (page 164), divided

1 garlic clove, minced

1 large egg, lightly beaten

2 tablespoons arrowroot starch, plus 4 teaspoons, divided

½ teaspoon dried thyme

¼ teaspoon ground nutmeg

1 teaspoon sea salt

Freshly ground black pepper

2 tablespoons ghee or avocado oil, divided

4 ounces button mushrooms, thinly sliced

2 cups Rich Chicken Broth (page 158) or store-bought chicken broth

FOR THE SALAD

2 tablespoons extra-virgin olive oil

1 tablespoon freshly squeezed lemon juice

4 cups baby spinach leaves

Sea salt

Freshly ground black pepper

1. **Prepare the steaks.** Combine the beef, pork, ¼ cup of caramelized onions, the garlic, egg, 2 tablespoons of arrowroot, the thyme, nutmeg, salt, and a few grinds of black pepper. Use your hands to gently combine, then form the mixture into 4 oblong patties.

2. **Fry the steaks.** Heat 1 tablespoon of ghee in a 12-inch skillet over medium-high heat. When the ghee is hot, add the steaks and fry until they are browned, about 5 minutes per side. Transfer the steaks to a platter and keep warm.

3. **Make the gravy.** Heat the remaining 1 tablespoon of ghee in the same pan over medium-high heat. When

the ghee is hot, add the mushrooms and a generous pinch of salt. Sauté the mushrooms, stirring up the browned bits, until lightly browned, about 4 minutes. In a medium bowl, whisk together the chicken broth and remaining 4 teaspoons of arrowroot until there are no lumps, then slowly whisk the mixture into the mushrooms. Stir the gravy until hot, clear, and thickened (do not boil). Remove the pan from the heat and stir in the remaining ¼ cup of caramelized onions. Season the gravy with salt and pepper. Return the steaks to the pan and spoon the gravy over them.

4. **Make the salad and serve.** In a small bowl, whisk together the olive oil and lemon juice. Divide the spinach among four dinner plates and drizzle the dressing over the spinach. Season with salt and pepper. Add a steak to each plate, top with the mushrooms and gravy, and serve.

SERVING SUGGESTION: Serve with mashed potatoes or mashed cauliflower.

Per Serving: *Calories: 489; Fat: 34g; Protein: 35g; Total Carbs: 12g; Fiber: 2g; Sodium: 856mg; Iron: 4mg*

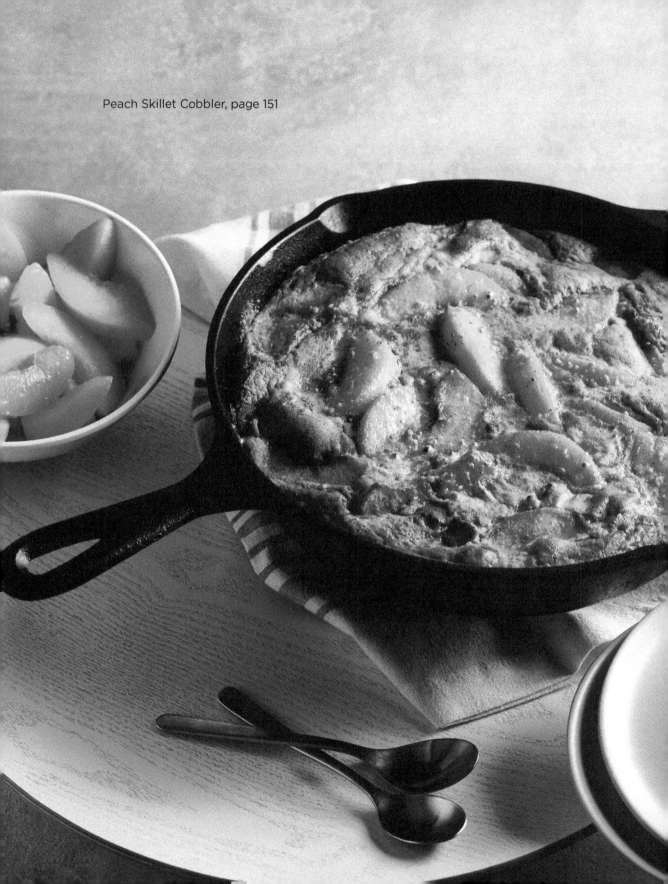

Peach Skillet Cobbler, page 151

CHAPTER EIGHT

Desserts

Almond Butter Chocolate Chip Cookies

Do you like your chocolate chip cookies crispy on the edges and chewy in the middle? That's how these turn out, all without butter or flour. For the most consistent results, look for no-stir almond butter. I've made these cookies with cashew butter as well, and they're just as delicious.

MAKES 16 COOKIES

Active time: 10 minutes
Total time: 20 minutes

....
LOW-CARB, VEGETARIAN

1 cup creamy no-stir almond butter

⅔ cup coconut sugar

1 large egg

1 teaspoon vanilla or almond extract

1 teaspoon baking soda

¼ teaspoon salt

½ cup coarsely chopped dark chocolate bar or Paleo chocolate chips

1. **Get ready.** Arrange two racks toward the center of the oven. Preheat the oven to 350°F. Line two rimmed baking sheets with parchment paper or aluminum foil.

2. **Make the dough.** In the bowl of a stand mixer, combine the almond butter, sugar, egg, vanilla, baking soda, and salt. Mix on low speed until well combined. Stir in the chocolate by hand.

3. **Bake the cookies.** Using a 2-tablespoon scoop, place 8 evenly spaced balls of dough on each baking sheet. Bake for 9 to 11 minutes, until the cookies are set and lightly browned. Place the baking sheets on wire racks. Let the cookies cool completely before removing them from the baking sheets. Store the cookies in a paper bag to keep them from becoming soft.

Per Serving *(1 cookie): Calories: 135; Fat: 10g; Protein: 4g; Total Carbs: 10g; Fiber: 2g; Sodium: 115mg; Iron: 1mg*

Individual Berry Granola Crisps

I wrote this recipe with frozen berries instead of fresh because they're terrific all year-round. If you use fresh berries, or even fresh peaches or cherries, decrease the time that the fruit bakes uncovered. To me, a crisp isn't a crisp without ice cream, so I'd suggest topping each ramekin with a scoop of coconut ice cream.

SERVES 4

Active time: 5 minutes
Total time: 30 minutes

....
5 INGREDIENTS, VEGAN

1 pound frozen berries, such as blueberries, raspberries, strawberries, and/or blackberries

2 tablespoons coconut sugar

1 tablespoon cassava flour

1 teaspoon ground cinnamon

1 cup Warm-Spice Granola (page 162) or store-bought Paleo granola

Vanilla coconut ice cream, for serving

1. **Get ready.** Preheat the oven to 375°F. Place 4 (6-ounce) ramekins on a rimmed baking sheet.

2. **Make the filling.** In a large bowl, combine the berries, sugar, flour, and cinnamon. Mix thoroughly. Divide the berries among the ramekins and bake for 15 to 20 minutes, until the berries are hot and bubbling. Remove from the oven.

3. **Finish the crisps and serve.** Divide the granola on top of the berry cups. Return to the oven and bake for 5 minutes. Cool for 5 minutes and serve warm, topped with ice cream.

Per Serving: Calories: 220; Fat: 11g; Protein: 4g; Total Carbs: 32g; Fiber: 3g; Sodium: 99mg; Iron: 1mg

Chocolate Avocado Pudding

This deceptively simple, no-cook recipe is packed with chocolatey goodness. You don't taste the avocado at all, it just imparts a wonderfully creamy texture. For a so-called dessert, this is very nutrient-dense and high in fiber. I don't know about you, but I'm willing to call this breakfast as well!

SERVES 4

Active time: 10 minutes
Total time: 10 minutes

....

5 INGREDIENTS, LOW-CARB, NO-COOK, NUT-FREE, ONE-PAN, SUPER FAST, VEGAN

2 medium ripe avocados, pitted and peeled

5 tablespoons unsweetened cocoa powder

6 tablespoons canned full-fat coconut milk, plus more as needed

4 tablespoons maple syrup, plus more as needed

1 teaspoon vanilla extract

Pinch sea salt

1. **Make the pudding.** Combine the avocado, cocoa, milk, maple syrup, vanilla, and salt in a blender. Blend until very smooth and creamy.

2. **Finish and serve.** Taste and adjust the sweetness by adding more maple syrup or adjust the consistency by adding more milk as needed. Serve.

SIMPLE SWAP: You can substitute honey for the maple syrup.

LOVE YOUR LEFTOVERS: Store leftover pudding in an airtight container in the refrigerator for up to 3 days or in the freezer for up to 1 month.

Per Serving: *Calories: 237; Fat: 16g; Protein: 4g; Total Carbs: 27g; Fiber: 9g; Sodium: 17mg; Iron: 2mg*

Peach Skillet Cobbler

Warm, juicy peaches under tender cake is my definition of summer perfection. This cobbler leans on nut butter for enough structure to be flourless. You can substitute honey for the maple syrup or use a combination of the two.

SERVES 8

Active time: 10 minutes
Total time: 30 minutes

....
VEGETARIAN

FOR THE BATTER

1 cup cashew butter

½ cup maple syrup

2 large eggs

½ teaspoon baking powder

¼ teaspoon sea salt

1 teaspoon vanilla extract

FOR THE COBBLER

1½ pounds ripe peaches, pitted and cut into ¼-inch slices

2 tablespoons coconut sugar

1 tablespoon cassava flour

1 teaspoon ground cinnamon

¼ teaspoon ground nutmeg

⅛ teaspoon ground cardamom

FOR SERVING

Vanilla coconut ice cream

1. **Get ready.** Preheat the oven to 375°F.

2. **Prepare the batter.** Combine the cashew butter, maple syrup, eggs, baking powder, salt, and vanilla in the bowl of a stand mixer. Mix on low speed until smooth. Set aside.

3. **Make the cobbler.** In a large bowl, toss the peaches with the sugar, flour, cinnamon, nutmeg, and cardamom. Pour the peaches into a 10-inch cast iron skillet. Pour the batter over the peaches and bake for 20 minutes, or until the top is set in the center and the peach juices are bubbling.

4. **Serve.** Spoon the cobbler into bowls and serve topped with coconut ice cream.

SIMPLE SWAP: You can substitute 1½ pounds frozen sweet cherries for the peaches. Add extra time if you don't thaw the cherries first.

Per Serving: *Calories: 313; Fat: 18g; Protein: 9g; Total Carbs: 32g; Fiber: 5g; Sodium: 20mg; Iron: 2mg*

Blueberry Mug Cake

If you have a blueberry muffin craving, this eggy mug cake will crush it. A mug cake is a single-serving cake mixed directly in a mug and then microwaved. I suggest blueberries here, but you could use raspberries, or go in a completely different direction and add Paleo chocolate chips or chopped dark chocolate. Don't fret if your cake collapses a bit into the mug—that's typical and the cake will still taste great.

SERVES 1

Active time: 5 minutes
Total time: 5 minutes

....

LOW-CARB, NUT-FREE, ONE-PAN,
SUPER FAST, VEGETARIAN

1 large egg

4 teaspoons avocado oil

1 tablespoon maple syrup

1 tablespoon coconut milk

1 teaspoon vanilla extract

4 teaspoons coconut flour

¼ teaspoon baking powder

Pinch sea salt

12 blueberries

1. **Make the mug cake.** In a microwave-safe coffee mug, combine the egg, oil, maple syrup, milk, and vanilla and whisk with a fork. Add the flour, baking powder, and salt and whisk until smooth. Stir in the blueberries.

2. **Cook and serve.** Microwave on high for 2 minutes. Add extra time in 10-second increments as needed. Serve warm.

SERVING SUGGESTION: A pat of ghee and a drizzle of maple syrup on top would be a wonderful way to gild the lily.

Per Serving: Calories: 375; Fat: 27g; Protein: 8g; Total Carbs: 25g; Fiber: 1g; Sodium: 78mg; Iron: 2mg

No-Bake Chocolate Crunch Cookies

The next time you're faced with a midafternoon slump, remember that you have a batch of these chewy-crunchy chocolate treats stashed in the refrigerator. A cross between a granola bar and a candy bar, these are a hit with everyone.

MAKES 24 COOKIES

Active time: 10 minutes
Total time: 30 minutes

5 INGREDIENTS, LOW-CARB, VEGETARIAN

¼ cup coconut oil or ghee

½ cup honey

¼ cup unsweetened cocoa powder

½ cup almond butter

1 teaspoon vanilla extract

¼ teaspoon sea salt

2 cups Warm-Spice Granola (page 162) or store-bought Paleo granola

1. **Prepare.** Line a rimmed baking sheet with parchment paper or aluminum foil.

2. **Make the cookies.** In a large saucepan, bring the coconut oil, honey, and cocoa powder to a boil over medium heat. Boil for 1 minute. Stir in the almond butter, vanilla, and salt. Add the granola and mix well. Drop cookies by the spoonful onto the prepared baking sheet.

3. **Finish and serve.** Freeze until firm, about 20 minutes. Serve cold.

SIMPLE SWAP: To make these cookies nut-free, make the granola with just seeds and use sunflower seed butter.

LOVE YOUR LEFTOVERS: Store the cookies in an airtight container in the refrigerator.

Per Serving (1 cookie): Calories: 132; Fat: 10g; Protein: 4g; Total Carbs: 9g; Fiber: 2g; Sodium: 27mg; Iron: 1mg

Mint Chocolate Chip Nice Cream

This quick dessert puts the creamy magic of frozen bananas to terrific use. Make sure the bananas are starting to have brown spots for the creamiest result. I love the addition of coconut cream—the solid cream in a can of full-fat coconut milk—for extra creaminess, but you can skip it if you'd like to keep the nice cream lighter.

SERVES 2

Active time: 5 minutes
Total time: 5 minutes

5 INGREDIENTS, NO-COOK, NUT-FREE, ONE-PAN, VEGAN

2 overripe bananas, peeled, halved, and frozen

¼ cup coconut cream

1 drop green natural food coloring (optional)

⅛ teaspoon real peppermint extract

Pinch sea salt

3 tablespoons Paleo chocolate chips or coarsely chopped dark chocolate

1. **Make the nice cream.** Combine the frozen bananas, coconut cream, food coloring (if using), peppermint extract, and salt in a blender. Blend, using a tamper if necessary, until completely smooth.

2. **Finish and serve.** Add the chocolate and blend briefly to break up the pieces a bit. Serve immediately.

Per Serving: Calories: 289; Fat: 17g; Protein: 3g; Total Carbs: 35g; Fiber: 5g; Sodium: 10mg; Iron: 5mg

Coconut Macaroons

This is a wonderful recipe for beginning bakers—even little ones can help measure ingredients and scoop the batter out. The only hard part is waiting for the macaroons to cool completely before digging in. There's no egg in this recipe and you won't miss it. In fact, the chewy, toasted coconut essence that makes macaroons so delicious is perhaps even more pronounced.

MAKES 24 MACAROONS

Active time: 15 minutes
Total time: 30 minutes

. . . .

5 INGREDIENTS, LOW-CARB, VEGETARIAN

1¼ cups unsweetened shredded coconut (not coconut chips or flakes)

¼ cup almond flour

¼ cup honey

3 tablespoons coconut oil

½ teaspoon vanilla or almond extract

⅛ teaspoon sea salt

1. **Get ready.** Arrange two oven racks toward the center of the oven. Preheat the oven to 350°F. Line two rimmed baking sheets with parchment paper or aluminum foil.

2. **Prepare the batter.** Pulse the coconut in a food processor until it is the texture of coarse sand. Add the almond flour, honey, coconut oil, vanilla, and salt and process until combined into a sticky batter.

3. **Bake the macaroons.** Use a 1-tablespoon scoop to portion out the macaroons, setting 12 on each prepared baking sheet. Bake for 12 minutes, or until golden brown. Cool completely on the baking sheets, then store in an airtight container.

SIMPLE SWAPS: To make vegan cookies, use maple syrup instead of honey. To make nut-free cookies, substitute cassava flour for the almond flour.

Per Serving *(1 macaroon): Calories: 58; Fat: 4g; Protein: <1g; Total Carbs: 6g; Fiber: <1g; Sodium: 26mg; Iron: <1mg*

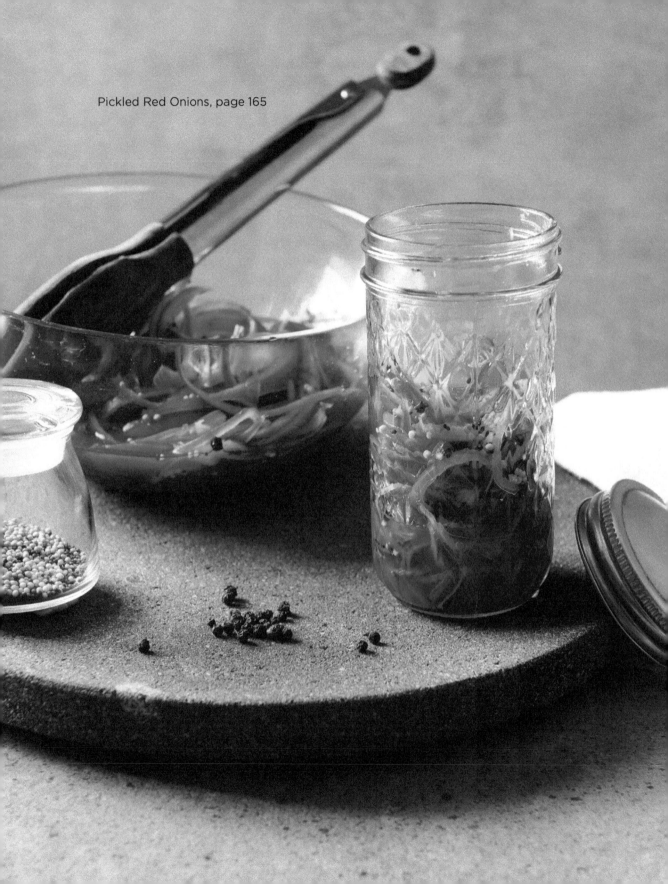
Pickled Red Onions, page 165

Condiments and Staples

Rich Chicken Broth

Chicken wings are easy to find, inexpensive, and make incredible broth. Hacking into the bones may seem like an unusual step, but it makes for extra rich and flavorful broth. This is a very pure chicken broth by design, so it can be used in a wide variety of recipes. This recipe takes longer than 30 minutes to prepare on the stovetop, but you can make it in 30 minutes using an Instant Pot or other pressure cooker.

MAKES ABOUT 8 CUPS

Active time: 15 minutes
Total time: 3 hours

5 INGREDIENTS, LOW-CARB,
NUT-FREE, ONE-PAN

2 pounds chicken wings

8 cups water

4 garlic cloves, smashed

2 bay leaves

1 medium yellow onion, quartered

1 teaspoon sea salt

1. **Prepare the chicken wings.** Lay the chicken wings on a cutting board and start hacking with your cleaver. Hack into the bones in a few places. If you hack all the way through the bone, that's okay. Toss the hacked pieces into a large stockpot. Add the water, garlic, bay leaves, onion, and salt.

2. **Simmer the broth.** Bring the broth to a very slow simmer over medium-low heat. Do not let it come to a full boil. When it's slowly simmering, turn the heat to low and let the broth barely simmer for 2 to 3 hours, skimming the top occasionally without stirring.

3. **Finish the broth.** Remove the pot from the heat and set aside until cool enough to handle. Set a colander in a large bowl and line the colander with two layers of cheesecloth. Strain the warm broth into the bowl. Discard the solids in the colander. Let cool, then store in an airtight container in the refrigerator for up to 3 days or in the freezer for up to 3 months.

Per Serving *(1 cup): Calories: 30; Fat: 1g; Protein: 4g; Total Carbs: <1g; Fiber: <1g; Sodium: 64mg; Iron: <1mg*

Plantain Tortillas

This recipe is the most popular recipe on my food blog, Fresh Tart. These tortillas are grain-free, nut-free, vegan, simple to make, and easy to freeze (I strongly suggest that you double the batch and freeze the extras)—and they're truly delicious. I use them for tacos, of course, but also for sandwiches and even as a hot dog "bun."

MAKES 12 TORTILLAS

Active time: 20 minutes
Total time: 30 minutes

. . . .
5 INGREDIENTS, LOW-CARB, NUT-FREE, VEGAN

1 pound large yellow (ripe) plantains, peeled and cubed

⅓ cup avocado oil

⅓ cup water

1 teaspoon sea salt

1. **Get ready.** Arrange two oven racks toward the center of the oven. Preheat the oven to 400°F. Line two rimmed baking sheets with parchment paper or aluminum foil.

2. **Make the batter.** Combine the plantains, oil, water, and salt in a blender and purée on the lowest setting for a minute or two. Gradually turn the speed up, using a tamper if needed to keep the purée moving around and adding a bit more water if absolutely needed, to form a thick, very smooth purée, similar in texture to smooth hummus.

3. **Make the tortillas.** Spoon the batter into 6 mounds on each prepared baking sheet and use a spoon or offset spatula to smooth them into rounds, about ¼ inch thick and 6 inches across. Bake for 10 minutes, switch racks, and bake for another 10 minutes, until just browning in spots. Cool for 5 minutes before serving.

COOKING HACKS: If you're extra pressed for time, spread the batter in one large, rectangular tortilla, dividing the batter between the two baking sheets. Bake and then cut each into 6 squares.

LOVE YOUR LEFTOVERS: Cool the tortillas to room temperature and store in an airtight container in the refrigerator for up to 3 days. Or, to freeze, stack the tortillas with squares of parchment paper between them and put them in a zip-top bag. To reheat from the refrigerator or freezer, gently warm in a skillet on the stovetop or in a toaster oven.

Per Serving *(1 tortilla): Calories: 96; Fat: 6g; Protein: <1g; Total Carbs: 12g; Fiber: <1g; Sodium: 93mg; Iron: <1mg*

Chimichurri

This version of chimichurri is based on arugula as well as fresh oregano. It's not traditional, but it comes together quickly and has a wonderful, peppery bite. I recommend doubling the recipe because you'll want extra on hand—it improves every meat and vegetable it touches and can stand in for a quick salad dressing.

MAKES 1 CUP

Active time: 5 minutes
Total time: 5 minutes
....
5 INGREDIENTS, LOW-CARB, NO-COOK, NUT-FREE, ONE-PAN, SUPER FAST, VEGAN

2 cups packed arugula leaves

2 tablespoons fresh oregano leaves

2 tablespoons chopped scallions, white and green parts

2 garlic cloves, chopped

½ cup extra-virgin olive oil

3 tablespoons red wine vinegar

½ teaspoon red pepper flakes

¾ teaspoon sea salt

Freshly ground black pepper

1. **Make the chimichurri.** Combine the arugula, oregano, scallions, garlic, olive oil, vinegar, red pepper flakes, salt, and black pepper in a blender and blend on medium speed until smooth, about 30 seconds. Taste and add more salt as needed.

2. **Store.** Keep in an airtight container in the refrigerator for up to 2 weeks.

Per Serving (1 tablespoon): Calories: 62; Fat: 7g; Protein: <1g; Total Carbs: <1g; Fiber: <1g; Sodium: 147mg; Iron: <1mg

Ginger-Scallion Sauce

This recipe is inspired by the food writer Francis Lam, who wrote a hilarious description of how to make the sauce, including to "salt the ginger and scallion like they called your mother a bad name." Even though the ginger and scallions are going into the food processor, cutting them into uniform pieces beforehand means you can achieve an even, fine mince without having to overprocess. As you will soon discover, this sauce tastes amazing on everything from eggs to pork to vegetables.

MAKES ABOUT 1½ CUPS

Active time: 10 minutes
Total time: 10 minutes

5 INGREDIENTS, LOW-CARB,
NUT-FREE, SUPER FAST, VEGAN

1 (2-ounce) piece fresh ginger, peeled and cut into ½-inch dice

2 bunches (8 ounces) scallions, white and green parts, cut into ½-inch pieces

Sea salt

¾ cup avocado oil

1. **Prepare the ginger and scallions.** In a food processor, process the ginger and scallions until finely minced but not puréed. Scrape into a large heat-proof bowl. Salt the ginger and scallions generously. You want it to be just a little too salty, to account for the oil.

2. **Finish the sauce.** Heat the oil in a small saucepan until shimmering. Drop a little piece of the ginger-scallion mixture in the oil to test the temperature—if it pops and sizzles, the oil is ready. Carefully pour hot oil into the ginger-scallion mixture. It will sizzle and bubble. Let cool to room temperature. Transfer to an airtight container and store in the refrigerator for up to 1 week.

Per Serving *(1 tablespoon): Calories: 125; Fat: 14g; Protein: <1g; Total Carbs: <1g; Fiber: <1g; Sodium: 194mg; Iron: <1mg*

Warm-Spice Granola

This crunchy, not-too-sweet, slightly salty granola makes a perfect breakfast, lunch, snack, or dessert. Now that's multitasking! Eat it by the handful, layer it with coconut yogurt or ice cream, or even press it into melted chocolate (perhaps with crumbled bacon?) for a quick bark. Many options, all of them delicious.

MAKES 6 CUPS

Active time: 10 minutes
Total time: 30 minutes

. . . .

LOW-CARB, VEGAN

2 cups unsweetened coconut flakes

2 cups sliced almonds

1 cup raw pepitas

½ cup sesame seeds

½ cup chopped raw cashews

½ cup maple syrup

2 tablespoons avocado oil

1 teaspoon vanilla extract

½ teaspoon ground cinnamon

⅛ teaspoon ground nutmeg

¾ teaspoon sea salt

1. **Get ready.** Preheat the oven to 300°F. Line a rimmed baking sheet with parchment paper or aluminum foil.

2. **Make the granola.** Combine the coconut, almonds, pepitas, sesame seeds, and cashews in a large bowl. In a small bowl, combine the maple syrup, oil, vanilla, cinnamon, nutmeg, and salt and stir to combine. Pour the oil mixture over the coconut mixture and toss to coat.

3. **Bake the granola.** Spread out the granola mixture on the prepared baking sheet. Bake for 10 minutes, stir, and bake for another 5 to 10 minutes, until nicely browned and crisp. Cool to room temperature (the glaze will harden) and store in an airtight container for up to 1 week.

SIMPLE SWAPS: To make nut-free granola, eliminate the almonds and cashews and use 2½ cups of coconut flakes, 2 cups of pepitas, and 1 cup of sunflower seeds.

Per Serving *(¼ cup): Calories: 135; Fat: 10g; Protein: 3g; Total Carbs: 11g; Fiber: 2g; Sodium: 97mg; Iron: 1mg*

Cashew Cheese

Cashews make a delicious purée on their own, but adding nutritional yeast is how you achieve a truly cheesy, umami flavor. Feel free to add any favorite soft herbs in place of or in addition to the chives. Basil, chervil, parsley, tarragon, or dill would be fantastic. This isn't a cheese that will "melt" in the traditional sense, so think of it more as a spread. For the best result, soak the cashews for 2 hours, but to make the recipe in less than 30 minutes, just skip the soak and blend the cashews as directed.

MAKES ABOUT 1 CUP

Active time: 5 minutes
Total time: 2 hours

. . . .

5 INGREDIENTS, LOW-CARB, NO-COOK, ONE-PAN, VEGAN

1 heaping cup raw cashews, soaked in water for at least 2 hours and drained

2 tablespoons minced fresh chives

1 small garlic clove, smashed

2 tablespoons nutritional yeast

2 tablespoons freshly squeezed lemon juice

½ teaspoon sea salt

Freshly ground black pepper

¼ cup water

1. **Make the cheese.** Combine the cashews, chives, garlic, nutritional yeast, lemon juice, salt, and a few grinds of pepper in a blender. Start blending on low and gradually turn up the speed to purée, using a tamper if needed. With the motor running, slowly drizzle in the water until the mixture is the consistency of a smooth, spreadable cheese. Taste and add more salt as needed, then purée again.

2. **Store.** Keep in an airtight container in the refrigerator for up to 1 week.

Per Serving *(1 tablespoon): Calories: 130; Fat: 10g; Protein: 5g; Total Carbs: 8g; Fiber: 1g; Sodium: 282mg; Iron: 2mg*

Caramelized Onions

You can't rush good caramelized onions. Keep a careful eye on them and stir frequently. If they are browning too fast, turn the heat down and/or add a bit of water to the pan. I especially love these in egg dishes and on top of burgers.

MAKES ABOUT 1 CUP

Active time: 1 hour
Total time: 1 hour

....

5 INGREDIENTS, LOW-CARB, NUT-FREE, ONE-PAN, VEGETARIAN

2 tablespoons ghee, avocado oil, or extra-virgin olive oil

2 large yellow onions, halved and thinly sliced

Sea salt

1 tablespoon balsamic vinegar or water

1. **Make the onions.** Heat the ghee in a large, heavy skillet over medium heat. When the ghee is hot, add the onions and a few large pinches of salt and stir to coat them in the oil. Sauté the onions, stirring every few minutes, until deeply browned, about 45 minutes. If the onions are browning too quickly, turn the heat down to medium-low. If the pan seems dry, add a bit more oil.

2. **Finish the onions.** When the onions are deeply browned, add the vinegar to deglaze the pan. Continue cooking until the liquid is absorbed. Season with additional salt. Cool to room temperature, then store in an airtight container in the refrigerator for up to 1 week.

Per Serving *(2 tablespoons): Calories: 47; Fat: 3g; Protein: <1g; Total Carbs: 4g; Fiber: <1g; Sodium: 147mg; Iron: <1mg*

Pickled Red Onions

The acidic zip and snap of pickled red onions is especially welcome in rich dishes like tacos, burgers, pizza, and creamy salads. Once you start to count on them, you'll want to have them on hand all the time. Luckily, they're a breeze to make and keep really well in the refrigerator.

MAKES 2 CUPS

Active time: 15 minutes
Total time: 15 minutes

5 INGREDIENTS, LOW-CARB, NUT-FREE, ONE-PAN, VEGAN

½ teaspoon black peppercorns

½ teaspoon mustard seeds

1 large red onion, very thinly sliced

½ cup apple cider vinegar

¼ cup water

1 teaspoon sea salt

2 tablespoons maple syrup

1. **Prepare the onions.** Put the peppercorns and mustard seeds in a pint-size glass jar. Add the onions. Set aside.

2. **Pickle the onions.** In a small saucepan, bring the vinegar, water, and salt to a simmer over medium heat. Remove from the heat and stir in the maple syrup. Pour the hot brine over the onions. Cool to room temperature and serve, or cover and refrigerate for up to 2 weeks.

Per Serving *(1 tablespoon): Calories: 6; Fat: <1g; Protein: <1g; Total Carbs: 1g; Fiber: <1g; Sodium: 73mg; Iron: <1mg*

Mayonnaise

A blender makes homemade mayonnaise super easy to make—and wow, does it taste amazing. Use where called for in the recipes in this book, as well as for dipping vegetables or topping burgers.

MAKES ABOUT 1 CUP

Active time: 5 minutes
Total time: 5 minutes

....

5 INGREDIENTS, LOW-CARB, NO-COOK, NUT-FREE, VEGETARIAN

1 large egg

4 teaspoons freshly squeezed lemon juice

1 teaspoon Dijon mustard

¼ teaspoon fine sea salt

¼ teaspoon freshly ground black pepper

1 cup avocado oil

1. **Make the mayonnaise.** Combine the egg, lemon juice, mustard, salt, and pepper in a blender and blend on medium speed until well combined. With the motor running, slowly drizzle the oil into the blender. As the emulsion comes together, keep adding the oil until it's all incorporated.

2. **Store.** Keep in an airtight container in the refrigerator for up to 1 week.

COOKING HACK: If you want to use an immersion blender, put the egg in the bottom of a pint-size jar. Top with the lemon juice, mustard, salt, and pepper. Pour the oil on last. Slowly insert an immersion blender, down to the bottom of the jar. Turn the blender on low speed and blend without moving the blender until the mixture starts to emulsify and turn white. Then slowly move the blender up and down a few times until the ingredients are well incorporated.

Per Serving *(1 tablespoon): Calories: 125; Fat: 14g; Protein: <1g; Total Carbs: <1g; Fiber: <1g; Sodium: 44mg; Iron: <1mg*

Measurement Conversions

	US STANDARD	US STANDARD (OUNCES)	METRIC (APPROXIMATE)
VOLUME EQUIVALENTS (LIQUID)	2 tablespoons	1 fl. oz.	30 mL
	¼ cup	2 fl. oz.	60 mL
	½ cup	4 fl. oz.	120 mL
	1 cup	8 fl. oz.	240 mL
	1½ cups	12 fl. oz.	355 mL
	2 cups or 1 pint	16 fl. oz.	475 mL
	4 cups or 1 quart	32 fl. oz.	1 L
	1 gallon	128 fl. oz.	4 L
VOLUME EQUIVALENTS (DRY)	⅛ teaspoon	———	0.5 mL
	¼ teaspoon	———	1 mL
	½ teaspoon	———	2 mL
	¾ teaspoon	———	4 mL
	1 teaspoon	———	5 mL
	1 tablespoon	———	15 mL
	¼ cup	———	59 mL
	⅓ cup	———	79 mL
	½ cup	———	118 mL
	⅔ cup	———	156 mL
	¾ cup	———	177 mL
	1 cup	———	235 mL
	2 cups or 1 pint	———	475 mL
	3 cups	———	700 mL
	4 cups or 1 quart	———	1 L
	½ gallon	———	2 L
	1 gallon	———	4 L
WEIGHT EQUIVALENTS	½ ounce	———	15 g
	1 ounce	———	30 g
	2 ounces	———	60 g
	4 ounces	———	115 g
	8 ounces	———	225 g
	12 ounces	———	340 g
	16 ounces or 1 pound	———	455 g

	FAHRENHEIT (F)	CELSIUS (C) (APPROXIMATE)
OVEN TEMPERATURES	250°F	120°C
	300°F	150°C
	325°F	180°C
	375°F	190°C
	400°F	200°C
	425°F	220°C
	450°F	230°C

Index

Acknowledgments

First of all, I'd like to thank all of the terrific and enthusiastic cooks and eaters (Nathan!) in my family. Despite being an incredibly picky eater as a child, the ritual of evening and holiday meals prepared at home from real-food ingredients is in my DNA. For that, I am lucky and grateful. No other life skill has served me so well.

Thank you also to my "foodist" friends here in Minneapolis/St. Paul, Minnesota. Twin Cities restaurants have come of age in the last decade, and I've been lucky to have one foot in that world. I've learned about technique, seasoning, and palate from many talented chefs and food-writer friends—in particular, the ladies of #L2!—and cooking with you all has been my joy.

I so enjoyed working with my editor, Natasha Yglesias of Callisto Media. It is a pleasure to have someone take your words and make you sound smarter and more concise than you are in real life. Thank you for considering me for this project and trusting me to provide helpful tips and delicious recipes for you all.

Adopting a Paleo lifestyle has transformed my health, so I want to send out a big thank you to the long-time Paleo and autoimmune protocol bloggers and writers who have helped so many people change their lives. It's hard to imagine that anyone thought that a diet of real, unprocessed food was a fad, but they did. Kudos to those of you who took the heat and kept writing anyhow.

And last, a giant shout-out to the recipe testers! Making the recipes in your busy home kitchens for people you love—there's no better test than that. Your feedback has been invaluable.

About the Author

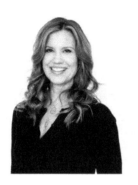

STEPHANIE A. MEYER is a Minneapolis-based author, recipe developer, health coach, and podcaster. She is the owner of Project Vibrancy Meal Plans and Coaching and writes the health food blog Fresh Tart. Meyer is also the creator of the Healing Green Broth 30-Day Challenge. Follow her on Instagram (@Stephanie.A.Meyer), and find her work and more recipes at StephanieAMeyer.com.

CPSIA information can be obtained
at www.ICGtesting.com
Printed in the USA
LVHW011453130220
646788LV00002B/3

9 781646 114788